Mourad Boukheloua
Souad Chelghoum

Cardio-renal syndrome :

Mourad Boukheloua
Souad Chelghoum

Cardio-renal syndrome :

at the crossroads of cardiology and nephrology

ScienciaScripts

Imprint

Any brand names and product names mentioned in this book are subject to trademark, brand or patent protection and are trademarks or registered trademarks of their respective holders. The use of brand names, product names, common names, trade names, product descriptions etc. even without a particular marking in this work is in no way to be construed to mean that such names may be regarded as unrestricted in respect of trademark and brand protection legislation and could thus be used by anyone.

Cover image: www.ingimage.com

This book is a translation from the original published under ISBN 978-620-3-45892-3.

Publisher:
Sciencia Scripts
is a trademark of
Dodo Books Indian Ocean Ltd. and OmniScriptum S.R.L publishing group

120 High Road, East Finchley, London, N2 9ED, United Kingdom
Str. Armeneasca 28/1, office 1, Chisinau MD-2012, Republic of Moldova, Europe
Printed at: see last page
ISBN: 978-620-6-22228-6

Foreword

After the hepato-renal syndrome and the pneumo-renal syndrome, a new syndrome involving close interaction between two noble organs - the heart and the kidney - has recently been described under the name of cardio-renal syndrome (CRS), defined by the expression of the mutual impact of the dysfunction of each organ.

Cardiac and renal pathologies taken in isolation are frequent, so their coexistence is not uncommon. Thus, CRS is an increasingly recognized diagnostic entity, albeit difficult to apprehend, with a non-negligible morbi-mortality compared to the tip of an iceberg hiding a host of dreadful complications.

New data on the pathophysiological mechanism have made it possible to better define the issue and optimize management with new therapeutic options.

In any case, cardio-renal syndrome is detrimental to health through its prognosis and to the state through its cost, and merits unceasing collaboration between the cardiologist and the nephrologist, the two pioneers who have the capacity for optimal management of such a scourge.

Mourad .BOUKHELOUA

Foreword

There are few textbooks describing cardio-renal pathology, and the interaction between these two noble organs and the difficulties involved in making diagnostic and therapeutic decisions prompted me and my cardiology colleague Prof. Mourad Boukheloua to publish this book.

A collaboration between cardiologists and nephrologists was born out of the need for each other's medical advice and the challenges encountered on a daily basis to optimize the management of patients with cardio-renal syndrome.

This manual is a review of recent literature, with a few illustrated real-life clinical cases, and is intended for: externs, medical interns, general practitioners and even specialists (cardiologists, nephrologists, internists, etc.), with the aim of raising awareness of this syndrome among the medical and paramedical professions.

In conclusion, I would like to dedicate this book to all my colleagues, residents and PhD students who work with patients with heart and kidney failure.

Souad Chelghoum

Abbreviations

Ag II: Angiotensin II
AHA: American heart association
ARB II: Angiotensin II receptor antagonist
ARNI: angiontensin receptor neprilysin inhibitor
AVP: Arginine/vasopressin
BNP: brain natriuretic peptide
CMD: dilated cardiomyopathy
COVID 19: coronavirus desease 19
CRP: C-reactive protein.
CRT: cardiac resynchronization therapy
ICD: implantable cardioverter defibrillator
LVAD: left ventricular assist device
eGFR: estimated glomerular filtration rate
T2DM: type 2 diabetes
RCT: randomized clinical trial
MRA: multicenter randomized trial
EER: extra-renal cleansing
LVEF: left ventricular ejection fraction
Hb: haemoglobin
HFpEF: heart failure with preserved ejection fraction
HFreEF: heart failure with reduced ejection fraction
HTA: high blood pressure
HD: hemodialysis
LVH: left ventricular hypertrophy
IC: heart failure
CHF: chronic heart failure
ICD: right heart failure
ACE inhibitor: ACE inhibitor
IL1: interleukin type 1
IL6: interleukin type 6
ARF: acute renal failure
CKD: chronic renal failure
MRI: magnetic resonance imaging
ESRD: end-stage renal disease

CVD: cardiovascular disease
NADPH: Nicotinamide Adenine Dinucleotide Hydrogen Phosphate
NT-proBNP: N terminal pro brain natriuretic peptide
NYHA: New York heart association
OD: right atrium
IAP: intra-abdominal pressure
PVC: central venous pressure
ROS: reactive oxygen species
ACS: acute coronary syndrome
CRS/RCS: cardio-renal/reno-cardiac syndrome
SGLT2: sodium/glucose transporter 2
S-ICD: subcutaneous implantable cardioverter defibrillator
SNS: sympathetic nervous system
RAAS: renin angiotensin aldosterone system
ST2: suppression of tumourigenicity 2
TAPSE: tricuspid annular plane systolic excursion
TNF a: tumor necrosis factor alpha
TWEAK: TNF-related weak inducer of apoptosis
LV/R: left/right ventricle

CONTENTS

I.   INTRODUCTION

Cardio-renal syndrome (CRS) is a term that generally refers to the collective dysfunction of the heart and kidneys, triggering a series of feedback mechanisms and resulting in damage to both organs.

The first mention of the term cardio-renal syndrome (CRS) dates back to the 2004 National Heart, Lung, and Blood Institute Task Force meeting to evaluate the interaction between the heart and kidneys, a term that refers to the dysfunction of the heart and kidney that causes a cascade of reactions that damage both organs (1).

While previously proposed definitions of CRS have focused on the cardiac impact of the disease on renal dysfunction, with heart failure (HF) being the archetypal cardiovascular disease that causes CRS renal dysfunction as a result of the various treatments administered to relieve the state of congestion secondary to heart failure, leading to a deterioration in renal function manifested by a reduction in GFR; a new, broader definition has recently been given: "a disorder of the heart or kidney in which acute or chronic dysfunction of one organ leads to acute or chronic dysfunction of the other".(1).

Although the term CRS is commonly used worldwide to refer to the pathophysiological interaction between two organs, a recent classification of CRS proposed by the 7th Acute Dialysis Quality Initiate consensus conference describes the syndrome as being divided into two categories: cardio renal syndromes, when cardiac dysfunction leads to renal dysfunction, and renocardiac syndromes, when primary renal dysfunction leads to cardiac dysfunction (1,2).

The pathophysiology of CRS involves multiple mechanisms (hemodynamic, neurohormonal, inflammatory and oxidative stress). In clinical practice, it is often difficult to identify the primary factor in organ dysfunction, especially when diabetes, hypertension and atherosclerosis affect the function of both organs, and causal relationships are not always obvious, with considerable overlap between these entities. (3).

It is important to understand the various mechanisms involved in the spread of this syndrome, given the aging of the population, longer cumulative exposure to common risk factors including hypertension, obesity, diabetes and vascular disorders, and advances in therapeutic management, equipment and devices enabling CI patients to improve their prognosis.   The prevalence of chronic kidney disease (CKD) and heart failure is likely to continue to rise (4,5).

II.   CLASSIFICATION

Based on pathophysiology, depending on the primary organ at the origin of dysfunction and the speed of acute or chronic onset, but also the presence of systemic disease affecting other organs besides the heart and kidney, five subtypes of this syndrome arise as shown in figure 1.

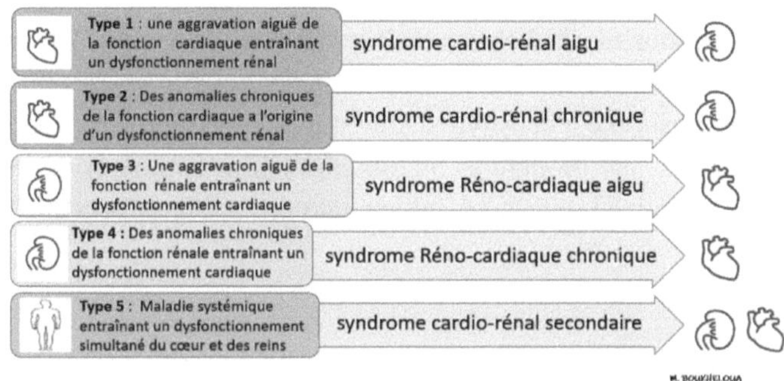

Figure 1Classification of cardio-renal syndrome. CRS has been subdivided into five types according to severity and order of organ involvement

SCR type I

Type I CRS is defined as an acute worsening of cardiac function leading to acute kidney injury (AKI), often as part of acute cardiac decompensation (40% of cases) with a mortality risk proportional to the degree of AKI, or cardiogenic shock secondary to acute coronary syndrome; on the other hand, prior CKD is a risk factor for type I CRS and predisposes to AKI in 60% of cases (1,2,4). Pathophysiologically,
this phenotype is characterized by hemodynamic compromise leading to hypoperfusion and congestion.

SCR type II

Type II CRS is characterized by a progression of CKD due to chronic decline in cardiac function; unlike Type I CRS, neurohormonal dysregulation, rather than hemodynamic impairment, is thought to play a central role in the pathophysiology of Type II CRS. CKD is common in patients with CHF, with more than half showing some degree of renal dysfunction; similar to type I CRS, in patients with systolic or diastolic CHF, the presence of renal failure is an independent negative prognostic factor (4).

SRC type III

Acute renal-cardiac syndrome is defined as the occurrence of acute cardiac injury in the setting of ARF. Prototypical situations include contrast-induced AKI, post-surgical AKI, glomerulonephritis, ischemia, rhabdomyolysis causing AKI and leading to acute heart failure; AKI can affect the heart acutely by multiple mechanisms, going beyond simple electrolyte disturbances and volume overload. These additional mechanisms are thought to be linked to an inflammatory flare-up and oxidative stress associated with AKI, which also adversely affect cardiac function (6).

Type IV CRS

Type IV CRS, also known as chronic renal-cardiac syndrome, is characterized by primary CKD leading to cardiac dysfunction and/or increased risk of adverse cardiovascular events (4) ; in a study by Cheung et al, up to 80% of patients with end-stage renal disease (ESRD) suffer from some form of cardiovascular disease, however, the prevalence of type IV CRS is more difficult to estimate, as it is often difficult to determine whether chronic renal dysfunction preceded cardiac disease or vice versa (7).

Uremic cardiomyopathy" has been implicated in type IV CRS, resulting from chronic uremic toxin and maladaptive neurohormonal balance causing chronic myocardial remodeling (8).

People with CKD face increased cardiac risk, with over 50% of deaths in stage V CKD patients attributed to CVD; after kidney transplantation, an increase in LVEF has been noted (3).

SRC type V

Type V or secondary CRS is characterized by the simultaneous development of cardiac and renal lesions caused by a systemic pathological process such as sepsis, autoimmune disease or hematological disease (9-11).

Recently, coronavirus (COVID-19) has received particular attention due to its association with acute multi-organ damage (12)The pathophysiology of type V CRS depends on the underlying disease and is often divided into acute and chronic type V CRS, with management generally aimed at treating the underlying disease process (antibiotics in sepsis, immunosuppression in lupus, chemotherapy in amyloidosis) and managing concomitant cardiac and renal damage.

III. ASSESSMENT OF CHANGES IN RENAL FUNCTION

Acute renal failure (ARF) refers to a sudden deterioration in renal function, leading to retention of extracellular volume, urea and other nitrogen toxins, with electrolyte disturbances.
Several consensus definitions of AKI have been established based on serum creatinine and urine output, but the most commonly used definition at present is the Improving Global Outcomes (KDIGO) kidney disease definition, essentially characterizing three categories as illustrated in Table 1 (13).

However, because of the volume expansion secondary to fluid retention in heart failure, there are doubts about the usefulness of creatinine as a diagnostic biomarker for ARF, since this value may be falsely normal or even low; on the other hand, an unmasked dilution effect may be falsely mistaken for ARF, leading to inappropriate discontinuation of diuretics, which would be deleterious in a patient with decompensated heart failure, causing an increase in morbidity and mortality.

Finally, there are a number of confounding situations, such as a rise in creatinine levels during treatment (33% of cases), which could even meet the KDIGO criteria for AKI, but is often referred to as a worsening of renal function, since it is a hemodynamic effect with no evidence of renal damage, at the same time, reduced muscle mass and protein intake, as well as increased levels of inflammation, modify creatinine levels, leading to errors in eGFR estimation (5).

CKD is defined by KDIGO as an abnormality of renal function (often defined by an eGFR below 60 ml/min/1.73 m2) or structure (albuminuria-although this may be due to cardiac dysfunction alone and not to CKD-, albumin/creatinine ratio > 30 mg/g, urine sediment abnormalities, tubular dysfunction, history of renal transplantation) that has been present for more than 3 months.

The recent KDIGO classification of CRS is based on glomerular filtration rate (GFR) and degree of albuminuria (A1<30 mg/g; A2 30-300 mg/g; A3>300 mg/g).

Stadium	Creatininemia	Diuresis
1	Elevation ≥ 3 mg/l Or 1.5-1.9 times base value	<0.5 ml/kg/h for 6-12h
2	2-2.9 times base value	<0.5 ml/kg/h for ≥12h
3	3 times base value Or Elevation ≥ 4 mg/l Or Initiation of renal replacement therapy Or In young people <18 years of age, a reduction in GFR to less than 35 ml/min/1.73 m² is recommended.	<0.3 ml/kg/h for ≥24 h Or Anuria for ≥ 12 h

Table 1: Stages of ARF according to KDIGO.

IV. PATHOPHYSIOLOGY

1. Role of central venous and intra-abdominal pressure

Intra-abdominal pressure (IAP) elevation, once observed and discussed in the context of surgical complications, is now increasingly recognized as an important pathophysiological contribution to CRS, since it can lead to intra-abdominal hypertension (IAP $\geq$12 mm Hg) at the origin of an abdominal compartment (IAP>20 mm Hg) in severe cases (14).

Acute cardiac decompensation leads to volume overload and increased central venous pressure, the latter attenuating the gradient and hence the flow of blood through the renal vasculature, and consequently to glomerular dysfunction with altered eGFR, decreased urine output and congestion (15).

In a study of 40 patients with acute cardiac decompensation, 60% had increased AIP with higher creatinine levels (2.3 1.0 mg/dL vs. 1.5 0.8 mg/dL; P 5 .009 respectively); their initiation of intensive medical treatment resulted in a significant reduction in right and left filling pressures and an improvement in cardiac index (CI), however these hemodynamic improvements were not correlated with improvements in renal function or PIA, but changes in PIA were correlated with changes in renal function. This disconnect between hemodynamics and AIP probably explains why a subset of patients show deterioration in renal function despite improvements in hemodynamics, because they show a persistent increase in AIP at follow-up (16).

On the other hand, a retrospective study of patients undergoing right heart catheterization showed that an increase in central venous pressure (CVP) above 6 mm Hg was associated with impaired renal function, thus emphasizing the close correlation between CVP and renal function, and its strong and independent predictive value of all-cause mortality (17).

In addition, a study of 196 heart failure patients showed that tricuspid regurgitation was independently associated with lower GFR by impeding venous return and reflux of blood into the renal-hepatic system(18).

2. Role of cardiac output and cardiac index

Initially, it was thought that the progressive impairment of renal function observed in heart failure was mainly due to poor renal perfusion secondary to low cardiac output, This hypoperfusion, perceived by the ascending branch of Henle's loop and the baroreceptors, leads to renin release from the juxtaglomerular cells of the afferent arterioles, resulting in sodium retention, increased vascular congestion and worsening renal function caused by vasoconstriction of the renal afferent arterioles.

Investigations suggest that the concept of managing CRS patients based solely on low-flow theory does not lead to improved outcomes; this suggestion is supported by the results of the ESCAPE (Evaluation Study of Congestive Heart Failure and Pulmonary Artery Catheterization Effectiveness) trial: a trial evaluating hemodynamic management of acute cardiac decompensation versus usual clinical care; among 433 people admitted with acute cardiac decompensation (cardiogenic shock state excluded), the investigators found no correlation between baseline renal function and CI; similarly, improvement in CI did not translate into improvement in renal function (19).

In contrast to these findings, a more recent study of patients in acute cardiogenic shock found an association between decreased CI and AKI, leading us to conclude that CI correlates with renal function but is not the only contributing hemodynamic process (20,21).

3. The role of neurohormonal dysregulation

In CHF, in order to restore tissue perfusion, neurohormonal mechanisms are activated, but their effect is often detrimental: firstly, the renin-angiotensin-aldosterone system (RAAS) plays an important role in the progression of renal lesions and the aggravation of CHF (22) secondly, the hyperactivity of the sympathetic nervous system (SNS) caused by impaired baroreceptors leads to increased renin release from the juxtamedullary cells of the kidney(23) the hydrostatic pressure detected in glomerular afferent arterioles, and the reduced amount of chloride delivered to the macula densa, result in increased renin levels, leading to excess synthesis of angiotensin II (Ang II), which has inappropriate systemic effects on the heart, vascular system and kidneys(24). In the kidneys,

Ang II causes an increase in sodium reabsorption (either indirectly, mediated by aldosterone, or by vasoconstriction of the renal efferent arteriole) and thus an increase in the fraction of renal plasma flow filtered through the glomerulus, which results in an increase in peritubular oncotic pressure and a lowering of hydrostatic pressure, or directly by sodium bicarbonate cotransporters in the proximal tubule and apical sodium-hydrogen exchangers,). Ang II also increases renal expression of endothelin-1 (ET-1) (25) a potent vasoconstrictor, pro-inflammatory and profibrotic peptide responsible for kidney damage; in the heart, ET1 induces cardiac myocyte hypertrophy via paracrine release of growth factor, and in the vascular system, it induces vascular smooth muscle contraction. In addition, Ang II mediates oxidative stress via the formation of reactive oxygen species (ROS) in cardiac and renal tissues, leading to inflammation and hypertension (26).

In IC patients, left ventricular dysfunction triggers activation of the SNS to maintain perfusion through mechanisms such as increased contractility, lusitropy and systemic vasoconstriction.

Adenosine is released in response to increased sodium load in the distal tubule and via type 1 adenosine receptors in the proximal tubule and afferent arterioles; it causes constriction of afferent arterioles and reduction of renal blood flow and GFR, while activation of adenosine type 2 receptors induces renin release and increases sodium reabsorption in the proximal tubule, reducing diuresis (27).

The efficacy of type 1 adenosine receptor antagonists in CRS is controversial, since the results of the PROTECT study (A Placebo-controlled Randomized Study of the Selective A1 Adenosine Receptor Antagonist Rolofylline for Patients Hospitalized with ADHF to Assess Treatment Effect on Congestion and Renal Function) showed that the rolofylline group failed to meet either primary (improvement in dyspnea) or secondary endpoints (death, cardiovascular or renal rehospitalization, or persistent renal failure); further clinical trials are therefore required   (28).
Arginine vasopressin (AVP) is a nanopeptide synthesized in the hypothalamus in response to serum osmolality; it is released in acute heart failure and induces water retention via vasopressin V2 receptors in the collecting duct; studies have shown that increased AVP levels contribute to the progression of CKD; the renal hemodynamic effects of AVP may be caused by its effects on the RAAS,

stimulating renin secretion directly via V2 activation or indirectly via reduced sodium concentration in the macula densa (29).

4.   The role of oxidative stress

Oxidative stress in CRS can be triggered by ischemic injury, venous congestion (which causes stress on endothelial cells) and inflammation; it is defined as an imbalance between oxidative and antioxidative factors, resulting in excessive accumulation of the former leading to cellular damage with ROS generation at mitochondrial level (30).

While most adenosine triphosphate (ATP) is produced by fatty acid oxidation in the heart, in heart failure there's a 30-40% drop in ATP synthesis as fatty acid oxidation shifts to glycolysis in myocytes to compensate for the energy deficit, but it remains insufficient to meet the energy needs of heart failure, generating a low threshold for hypoxemia, apoptosis and cell death.

In one study, patients admitted with acute cardiac decompensation who subsequently developed ARF were investigated for markers of oxidative stress (IL6, myeloperoxidase, nitric oxide, copper/zinc superoxide dismutase and endogenous peroxidase). Results showed a significantly higher presence of both oxidative stress markers in patients who developed type 1 CRS with lipotoxicity secondary to the accumulation of free fatty acids through reduced mitochondrial oxidative metabolism (31).

In addition to the deleterious effects of volume expansion and hemodynamics, RAAS and SNS activation also play an important role in amplifying oxidative stress in patients with CI and CKD.

Ang II has a deleterious effect by activating NADPH-oxidase in endothelial cells, renal tubular cells and cardiac myocytes, promoting oxidative damage by producing ROS causing mitochondrial dysfunction (32,33).

Patients with advanced CKD and end-stage renal disease (ESRD) present certain factors, such as uremic toxins and the dialysate solutions used in renal replacement therapy, which could lead to increased synthesis and release of pro-inflammatory cytokines, oxidative stress, immune system dysregulation leading to carotid artery intima-media thickening (a marker of early atherosclerosis) and left ventricular hypertrophy. Patients with ESRD have a higher cardiovascular morbidity and mortality that cannot be explained by conventional cardiac risk factors, namely, oxidative stress, endothelial dysfunction and hyperhomocysteinemia may play an additive role in these patients (34).

5.   Role of inflammatory mediators

CKD and CI are states of increased chronic inflammation, leading to the production of pro-inflammatory biomarkers (cytokines such as TNF-a and TWEAK, members of the IL-1 family, and IL-6), triggered by SNS, RAAS, venous congestion, ischemia and oxidative stress, implicated in tissue damage, fibrosis and apoptosis in both organs.

In the kidney, TNF-a and IL-6 increase the expression of monocyte chemoattractant proteins, promoting the accumulation of inflammatory cells in the interstitium. TNF-a also induces glomerular damage through apoptosis of mesangial cells. We also cite soluble ST2, an IL-1 family member with prognostic value for all-cause mortality in patients with CHF(35) levels of these pro-inflammatory markers have also been shown to be higher in people with CKD or on dialysis (36).

C-reactive protein (CRP), an acute-phase reagent, contributes to the pathogenesis of atherosclerosis by activating the complement system and stimulating the production of tissue factor (a potent procoagulant) by monocytes (37).

In a study of 4,269 people hospitalized for acute CHF, patients with CRP in the fourth quartile (9.6 mg/L) were independently associated with higher mortality (adjusted hazard ratio, 1.68) within 120 days of hospital discharge (38). In hemodialysis patients, elevated CRP levels predict left ventricular dysfunction, cardiac hypertrophy and mortality; these inflammatory proteins are not simply inert markers of disease activity, but play an active and complex role in the pathophysiology of CRS (39).

6.   Role of disturbances associated with renal failure

Protein-bound uremic toxins (PBUTs) are currently a new area of interest due to their potential association with cardiovascular disease. Indoxyl sulfate (IS) and p-cresyl sulfate (PCS) are the two most extensively studied uremic toxins that have been shown to play a role in the pathogenesis and progression of CRS through altered oxidative stress, endothelial dysfunction, impaired LV diastolic function, atherosclerosis, nephrotoxicity, reduced endothelial proliferation, impaired wound repair, and cardio-renal fibrosis, suggesting their role in the progression of CKD(40-42)A study of 139 CKD patients showed that IS was a powerful predictor of overall and cardiovascular mortality (43).

Fibroblast growth factor 23 (FGF23), a hormone produced in bone that controls phosphate and vitamin D metabolism by the kidneys, is an important predictor of adverse cardiovascular outcomes in patients with CKD and ESRD, since the increase in this factor has been associated with left ventricular hypertrophy through impaired ventricular contractility and relaxation (although this remains debatable due to the absence of alpha-klotho receptors that mediate FGF23 action in the heart), greater rhythmic risk through altered calcium membrane permeability has been reported with higher mortality in patients with advanced CKD (44).

7.   Role of anemia

Anemia is common in patients with CKD and CI, and is associated with cognitive impairment with poor quality of life, progression of renal disease, cardiovascular comorbidities and higher mortality; with a prevalence between 5% and 55% in CRS, it is considered an independent predictor of mortality (45). In the OPTIMIZE-HF (Organized Program to Initiate Lifesaving Treatment in Hospitalized Patients With Heart Failure) study of over 48,000 patients, 51.2% had mild anemia (hemoglobin level <12.1 g/dL) and 25% were moderately to severely anemic (hemoglobin level 5 to 10.7 g/dL) (46). In another multicenter study of 5222 CKD patients, 47.7% were anemic (hemoglobin level 12 g/dL) (47).

Anemia contributes to the pathophysiology of CRS in several ways: hypoxia on an already stressed heart or diseased kidney can induce ischemic threats that can lead to progressive cell death in both organs; red blood cells contain many antioxidants, so anemia can lead to increased oxidative stress, tissue ischemia and peripheral vasodilatation, leading to activation of the SNS, RAAS, and release of antidiuretic hormone, resulting in vasoconstriction, water and salt retention, and chronic renal venous congestion leading to nephron loss and interstitial fibrosis (48).

Chronic anemia also leads to left ventricular hypertrophy and myocardial cell death through ischemia and necrosis (49).

While correction of anemia in CHF patients with erythropoiesis-stimulating agents is beneficial (reduced hospitalization, improved New York Heart Association class, 6-minute walk test and quality of life), but normalization of hemoglobin levels may be deleterious, since trials targeting higher hemoglobin levels (13 g/dL) were paradoxically associated with a higher rate of adverse events (50).

The TREAT (Trial to Reduce Cardiovascular Events with Aranesp Therapy) study was a randomized, double-blind, placebo-controlled trial involving over 4,000 patients, the use of darbepoetin alfa in patients with diabetes, CKD and moderate anemia who were not going to benefit from dialysis to achieve an Hb target of 13 g/dl, showed no reduction in the risk of death, cardiovascular event or renal event, but rather an increased risk of fatal or non-fatal stroke in patients in the darbepoetin alfa group (51).

The REDHF (Reduction of Events by Darbepoetin Alfa in Heart Failure) study was a randomized, double-blind trial involving 2,278 systolic heart failure patients with mild to moderate anemia (hemoglobin level, 9.0-12.0 g/dL), patients were randomized to receive either darbepoetin alfa (to achieve a target hemoglobin level of 13 g/dL) or placebo, there was no difference in primary outcome (death from any cause or hospitalization for worsening CHF) (52).

Anemia plays an important role in the pathophysiology of CRS, and the management of anemia is complex, particularly in patients with CKD and CHF; the main unanswered question is the range of hemoglobin levels to aim for in this population (targets based on CKD guidelines:10-12 g/dL, or higher:12-13 g/dL but lower than 13 g/dL -because trials with hemoglobin levels of 13 g/dL or higher have been associated with negative results-).

8.   Pathogenesis of type 5 cardio-renal syndrome

CRS-5 has been classified into four stages: superacute, acute, subacute and chronic; systemic diseases likely to lead to CRS-5 include sepsis, connectivites such as lupus, sarcoidosis, amyloidosis and cirrhosis ; renal and cardiac damage is often mediated by pro-inflammatory cytokines, complement factors and RAAS activation, which are often the common terminal pathway in other forms of CRS, e.g. in sepsis, early increases in renal vascular resistance, pro-inflammatory cytokines (IL-6) and oxidative stress can lead to organ damage. Sepsis also leads to autonomic nervous system dysfunction and activation of the RAAS (53) the multitude of effects of sepsis on the function of various organs, including the heart and kidneys, makes it difficult to differentiate between the effects of sepsis and those of disease.   In addition, the management of sepsis can contribute to the development of CRS-5: fluid restoration can lead to tissue edema, increased venous congestion and reduced renal perfusion, iodinated contrast agents and certain drugs can lead to myocardial dysfunction and nephrotoxicity, resulting in the onset and/or worsening of CRS-5. In chronic inflammatory and autoimmune disease processes, the concomitant damage to both organs and the permanent interdependence between the heart and kidney lead to a pathophysiological mechanism similar to that discussed in other types of CRS (54).

9.   Future prospects

Understanding of the pathophysiology of CRS is not yet sufficient for optimal therapeutic control in these patients, due to a lack of precision in the diagnosis of AKI based on conventional biomarkers such as creatinine, which should give way to new filtration markers, such as cystatin C, beta-2 microglobulin and beta-trace protein, and to more sensitive, or even specific, tubular markers (55).

V.   DIAGNOSTIC

1.   Biological markers

The diagnosis of CRS requires the presence of signs and symptoms of CHF, as well as evidence of a structural or functional abnormality of the heart and kidneys.

Among cardiac biomarkers, we cite BNP and NT- proBNP, which are markers of myocardial stretching with value

diagnostic and prognostic in acute and chronic IC, with significantly greater BNP elevation in SCR than in patients with acute IC without renal failure (8).

In a study of 720 patients with acute IC by van Kimmenade et al. the combination of high NT-proBNP and eGFR<60 ml/min/1.73 m² was predictive of 60-day mortality (odds ratio 3.26), while NT-proBNP below the median was not associated with reduced 60-day survival, irrespective of impaired renal function at presentation or onset of renal failure at admission, indeed, lowering NT-proBNP levels during treatment of acute CHF was associated with improved outcomes, even in patients with a decline in renal function during treatment (56,57).

It has also been shown that in acute CHF, an elevated ratio of NT-proBNP to BNP precedes the onset of acute renal failure, providing another potential new parameter for risk stratification and prediction of CRS.

In addition to traditional cardiac biomarkers, other biomarkers such as galectin-3, ST2 (tumorigenicity suppressor), angiotensin-converting enzyme and PENK (proenkephalin A) have been investigated as novel markers of cardiac dysfunction, although they are not yet validated at present (58,59).

Renal biomarkers.

Although the current definition of ARF in clinical practice is based on changes in serum creatinine or urine output, these parameters reflect the filtration function of the kidneys and are relatively late findings in the development of ARF; in addition, other causes of creatinine elevation such as sarcopenia (which affects up to 20% of patients with chronic heart failure(60)); hence the focus on Cystatin C, a small 13 kDa protein of greater interest in elderly patients with wasting skeletal muscle suffering from CHF and other comorbidities, since it is less influenced by body composition and other non-renal factors such as age and gender (61)it is produced at a constant rate and is freely filtered in the glomerulus, without tubular secretion, and therefore a sensitive marker of eGFR and earlier AKI with prognostic value as an indicator of pre-hospitalization and mortality in patients with acute heart failure, albeit with less precise diagnostic value (62).

Several new renal biomarkers of tubular damage have been identified and could enable earlier diagnosis of AKI, although they have not yet been validated and are still under investigation: IGFBP-7 (Insulin-like growth factor-binding protein 7), TIMP-2 (tissue inhibitor of metalloproteinase-2), NGAL (Neutrophil Gelatinase-Associated Lipocalin), KIM-1 (Kidney injury molecule-1), in parallel other biomarkers involved in fibrosis may help determine the chronicity of renal dysfunction.

Urinalysis

Albuminuria informs us about glomerular function and integrity in CRS, even though it may be secondary to diabetes, hypertension or another renal problem, and has prognostic value for all-cause mortality, cardiovascular mortality and readmission in patients with CHF apart from GFR and other cardiovascular risk factors, as shown in substudies of the CHARM, GISSI-HF and Val-HeFT trials(63). In CRS, to counteract renal hypoperfusion there is hydrosodium retention through neurohormonal activation; although interpretation of natriuresis may prove difficult, particularly when diuretics are used, its prognostic value in CRS patients is certain, indeed Martens et al. have shown that among patients with stable CHF, those who subsequently developed CHF had lower natriuresis, with an acute fall in the week before hospitalization.

This finding was supported by the IMPROVE-HF trial of patients with IC and renal dysfunction, where urinary sodium at presentation was inversely related to 24-hour diuretic efficacy (64).

2. Imaging

Certain hemodynamic parameters easily obtained by transthoracic echocardiography are independently associated with a higher incidence of CRS (acute and chronic forms) such as elevated central venous pressure and filling pressures or decreased cardiac output and LVEF, the latter being an independent predictor of worsening renal function in patients hospitalized for acute IC (65).

Decreased (TAPSE), a surrogate for VD function, strongly predicts the development of acute CRS in patients with inferior wall ACS (66). Other common parameters include the ratio of mitral flow velocity to early diastolic mitral annular velocity, or E/E' ratio, to assess impairment of diastolic function (67).

Speckle echocardiography with strain analysis is an emerging quantitative technique that allows more accurate and early assessment of altered myocardial systolic function. Left ventricular longitudinal strain is significantly reduced in CKD despite preserved LVEF, providing a potential method of early detection of uremic cardiomyopathy (68).

Intrarenal Doppler ultrasonography to assess intrarenal hemodynamics has prognostic value in patients with heart failure; intrarenal venous flow, being correlated with DO pressure and thus renal congestion, predicts cardiovascular mortality and hospitalization for CHF at 1 year, independent of other risk factors; on the other hand, the renal venous stasis index and the integral of renal artery flow velocity are associated with the development of ARF in acute CHF and the increased rate of adverse cardiac events, respectively (69).

Renal ultrasonography is also useful for identifying chronic renal dysfunction in CRS and excluding other etiologies of AKI such as postrenal obstruction.

MRI offers an unrivalled assessment of ventricular dimensions and myocardial function, and also highlights myocardial fibrosis and inflammation, helping to identify possible systemic causes of myopathy; despite the limitations of its use in advanced CKD, a recent study has shown the usefulness of non-contrast native T1 relaxation time and global longitudinal strain as markers of fibrosis and myocardial dysfunction in hemodialysis patients (70).

Renal MRI provides a better understanding of the pathogenesis of CRS. To distinguish the chronic from the acute, Breidthardt's team focused on renal T1 relaxation time, which would be prolonged in isolation without indices of renal cortical perfusion (71).

3.   Blood volume assessment

Management of the SCR involves meticulous management of blood volume to improve congestion. Nevertheless, assessment of volumetric status based solely on clinical evaluation is imprecise; for this purpose, the gold standard is right heart catheterization, but this is criticized for being invasive. (72)It is a class 2a recommendation for cardio-renal patients in the AHA guidelines on CI (63); in parallel, new hemodynamic parameters, such as the pulmonary artery pulsatility index (PAPi) and the DO/pulmonary capillary pressure ratio, which reflect LV dysfunction, have also proved useful for predicting renal dysfunction in patients with CI (73,74).

VI. SPECIAL FEATURES

1. Heart failure with preserved ejection fraction

Nearly 50% of heart failure patients have a preserved ejection fraction; it's important to understand the renal consequences of HFpEF, in heart failure patients, it has been shown that AKI and advanced CKD are independent predictors of in-hospital mortality.   Elevated central venous and intra-abdominal pressure, left ventricular hypertrophy, left ventricular deformation, RAAS activation, valvulopathies, oxidative damage and the role of pulmonary hypertension and autonomic respiratory system dysfunction play a key role in the pathogenesis of the cardio-renal syndrome in the context of HFpEF. A good understanding of the hemodynamic factors involved in this interface between CI and renal failure is essential to provide optimal decongestant therapies as well as targeted medical treatment of the cardio-renal syndrome.

Finally, new targeted therapies such as the development of angiotensin/neprilysin inhibitors and SGLT-2 inhibitors offer new prospects for reducing the adverse effects of HFpEF in this population. Future studies focusing exclusively on renal outcomes in patients with HFpEF are crucial to providing optimal therapies for this patient subgroup. To this end, the availability of biomarkers of renal and cardiac injury offers a new dimension for the accurate diagnosis and quantification of end-organ damage in HFpEF and will improve the accuracy of goal-directed therapies in this population (75).

2. Right heart failure and cardio-renal syndrome

Traditionally, the causes of CRS have been attributed to renal hypoperfusion resulting from low cardiac output and excessive diuresis; however, in recent decades, evidence has increasingly demonstrated a correlation between venous congestion and CRS, rather than low cardiac output, linking the failing right heart to CRS.
Systemic venous congestion develops in the context of DCI - often the final pathway of many cardiovascular diseases - which can be seen in either isolated VD or biventricular failure.

The consequences of venous congestion on various organs (retrograde congestion) play a central role in the pathophysiology of CRS and have both local (renal and splanchnic congestion) and systemic effects at the origin of mechanical, biological and immune responses, which contribute to the development of CRS, firstly through elevated renal venous pressure that obliterates renal tubules by distending renal venules (76) reducing renal perfusion pressure (RPP) and by increasing renal interstitial pressure through fluid extravasation, leading to a hypoxic state of the renal parenchyma and tubular dysfunction, but also through activation of the RAAS, SNS and vascular inflammation through endothelial cell dysfunction at the origin of veno-lymphatic congestion of the abdominal organs (77,78).

Right ventricular dilatation and dysfunction as a result of elevated filling pressures leads to a leftward displacement of the interventricular septum with changes in LV geometry, resulting in lower preload and cardiac output, thus reducing renal arterial pressure; recent data have shown a greater correlation between venous congestion and renal dysfunction, representing the significant influence of the right heart, so its assessment and parallel monitoring of renal function by known and emerging tools such as renal Doppler ultrasound or new biomarkers may have direct clinical implications; finally, decongestion remains the basic strategy in this situation (79).

3. Preeclampsia: a cardio-renal syndrome during pregnancy

In cardiac terms, pre-eclamptic pregnancies are characterized by eccentric and concentric remodeling of the left ventricle (LV), with impaired contractility and diastolic dysfunction (80). Left atrial size is increased, accompanied by elevated levels of atrial natriuretic peptide (ANP), and there is global systolo-diastolic dysfunction of the right ventricle. Renal lesions associated with preeclampsia include proteinuria and its pathological substrates, endotheliosis (loss of capillary space and obliteration of endothelial fenestrons) and/or thrombotic microangiopathy. Renal lesions have been linked to deficiency of vascular endothelial growth factor (81) and to the loss of glomerular epithelial cells (i.e., podocytes) and/or the depletion of podocyte-specific proteins and the consequent disruption of the tight junctional barrier (82).

The clinical presentation of renal and cardiac abnormalities in preeclampsia is multifaceted and can be interpreted in the context of CRS subtypes.
Pre-eclampsia most closely resembles CRS type 5: it is characterized by simultaneous dysfunction of the heart and kidneys, leading to a vicious circle of worsening cardiac and renal function and clinical signs and symptoms that are common to both conditions.

The systemic nature of the disease is linked to several pathogenic mechanisms common to both pre-eclampsia and CRS type 5; these include activation of the sympathetic nervous system, neurohormonal stress, inflammation, hemodynamic changes, hypoxia, oxidative stress and increased renal vascular resistance, leading to activation and induction of cytokines, leukocytes and Toll-like receptors (77).

Pre-eclampsia may initially present as type 1 CRS, with hypertensive pulmonary oedema, preserved left ventricular function and accompanying acute renal injury, or type 3 CRS, with hypertension and acute renal injury, ultimately leading to acute cardiac decompensation. In addition, cardiac damage and hypertension may occur during pregnancy in the context of previous proteinuric renal disease (not always diagnosed prior to pregnancy), ultimately leading to clinical features of preeclampsia. The temporal sequence, i.e. CKD before pregnancy, may be consistent with type 4 CRS, in which the hemodynamic changes of pregnancy and increased circulating plasma volume, in particular, may unmask and exacerbate underlying endothelial dysfunction, leading to hypertension and cardiac dysfunction. Whatever the presentation
(CRS type 1, type 2 or type 4), preeclampsia in general, and its early, severe forms, tend to progress rapidly to systemic disease and CRS type 5 (83).

Finally, type 2 CRS can occur in pregnant women with pre-pregnancy heart disease, as these women are at increased risk of cardiovascular and systemic complications. In the absence of pre-existing hypertension, these women rarely present with the clinical features of pre-eclampsia.

4.   Type 2 diabetes and cardio-renal syndromes

In a national study involving over 5 million patients, it was found that around 80% of patients had died after 5 years' follow-up. This mortality rate is very high and underlines that CKD and CI are very serious conditions, particularly in elderly populations with severe comorbidities; on the other hand, it was found that patients with T2DM account for almost half of CRS patients, and that these syndromes occur at a younger age in diabetic patients. The prognosis of CRS is poor, even more so in patients with T2DM, the latter as such increasing the risk of death, cardiovascular events and end-stage renal failure, but not ischemic stroke. The mechanisms linking diabetes and CRS are incompletely understood. These data broaden the scope of T2DM complications and provide further evidence for the compelling need for primary and secondary prevention of renal and cardiovascular complications in people with T2DM on the basis of research transcending traditional specialty boundaries (84).

5.   A new approach to pediatric cardio-renal syndrome

The case of an adolescent with a cardio-renal syndrome due to advanced chronic kidney disease with severe secondary heart failure was studied, where a joint kidney and heart transplant was initially considered due to the severity of his cardiac dysfunction.

During transplant evaluation, he was treated with a strategy of intermittent hemodialysis combined with peritoneal dialysis; subsequently his hemodynamics improved to the point that he was able to undergo renal transplantation alone, followed by a rapid improvement in his cardiac function, which completely normalized within 6 weeks of renal transplantation, enabling successful renal transplantation alone and avoidance of cardiac transplantation ; combined dialysis is an uncommon and previously unreported strategy for cardiac rehabilitation and the avoidance of multi-organ transplantation in paediatric patients, thus preserving the allocation of cardiac transplant resources to those who need them most (85).

VII. SCR MANAGEMENT AND SUPPORT

1.   Congestion therapy

Diuretics. Hypoperfusion and, above all, congestion both play an important role in renal dysfunction in acute and chronic CI, which is why diuretics are the cornerstone of management of these patients, even if this is purely symptomatic treatment with no proven benefit in terms of mortality or rehospitalization.

Loop diuretics are the main class of diuretics, and include furosemide, bumetanide, torsemide and ethacrynic acid; while thiazide-type diuretics augment the response to loop diuretics in cases of diuretic resistance.

Several studies have evaluated different dosing protocols, the largest to date being the DOSE-AHF trial, which randomized 308 patients with acute IC to bolus or continuous infusion of low- or high-dose furosemide; in the latter category, secondary endpoints (dyspnea, net fluid loss and weight loss at 72 hours) were improved with fewer side effects, while there were no significant differences in symptoms or renal function (86).

Based on the DOSE-AHF, CARRESS-HF and ROSE-AHF studies, and a meta-analysis of randomized controlled trials (RCTs) evaluating the efficacy of continuous infusion versus bolus injection of loop diuretics (87,88)The results: aggressive diuresis appears to be conducive to rapid improvement of acute CHF symptoms and is not associated with an increased risk of renal dysfunction, even though the latter may worsen early in the course of treatment; rates of cardiovascular death or hospitalization for cardiovascular or renal reasons remain similar to those of patients whose renal function has not deteriorated, as long as patients show a good diuretic response to continuous infusion. In patients with diuretic resistance, very high doses of diuretics are required and, in practice, many patients prefer continuous infusion to boluses, which can exceed >200 mg furosemide in cases of severe resistance.

In a post-hoc analysis of the CARRESS-HF trial, it was observed that intensive volume removal led to a further increase in creatinine in around half of patients with acute IC whose renal function was already worsening (89).

Patients with increased biomarkers of tubular injury in response to intensive volume removal had better decongestion and paradoxically better creatinine recovery at 60 days, providing further support for intensive volume removal (74).

Urinary sodium analysis after initial diuresis may be useful in predicting response to diuretics. In a study using the furosemide stress test protocol (1 mg/kg for loop diuretic-naive patients or 1.5 mg/kg for loop diuretic-experienced patients as the initial dose) for patients with acute heart failure, urinary sodium >83 mmol/L 2 h after the initial dose had a sensitivity of 96% to predict a 30% reduction in NT-proBNP on day five (90).

A scenario clinicians are often faced with concerns the use of diuretics in a hypotensive patient who is obviously congested. Although the common misconception is not to administer diuretics for fear of worsening hypotension, the presence of hypotension in a congested patient is a sign of a very ill patient in need of urgent aggressive decongestion and simultaneous blood pressure support with vasoactive therapies. The idea of ventricular interdependence postulates that right ventricular volume or pressure overload leads to a decrease in left ventricular filling due to forces directly transmitted from one ventricle to the other, so in the setting of simultaneous congestion and hypotension, decongestion of the VD can lead to a decrease in ventricular interdependence, thereby improving LV filling and increasing cardiac output and blood pressure (79).

In an ancillary ROSE-AHF study that measured biomarkers of renal damage (NGAL, NAG, KIM-1) in patients undergoing aggressive diuresis, worsening renal function in the context of aggressive diuresis was not associated with an increase in biomarkers of tubular damage; overall, it has been suggested that impaired renal function in itself is not the main determinant of outcome, and that the context in which it develops may be more clinically relevant (91).
The optimal diuretic strategy is expected with the ongoing PUSH-AHF and ENACT-HF studies, which incorporate natriuresis-guided therapy in patients with acute-phase IC, whereas in cases of severe renal dysfunction, further studies are needed (92).

Ultrafiltration. Veno-venous ultrafiltration, also known as aquapheresis, is an alternative decongestion method for patients with acute CHF and CRS, involving the passage of blood through a semi-permeable material to remove isotonic fluids from the intravascular space, a fairly practical technique, especially with the development of simplified peripherally-inserted ultrafiltration systems requiring minimal operator intervention, allowing greater control over the rate and volume of fluid removal, less neurohormonal activation, greater net sodium loss and the possibility of avoiding worsening renal function in patients with CRS (93).

Several studies have examined the effects of ultrafiltration versus diuretic therapy in acute CHF, with somewhat variable results, we cite the landmark CARRESS-HF trial which is the only one to have examined patients with acute type I CRS, the trial randomized 188 patients with acute CHF and worsening renal function, Here, ultrafiltration proved inferior to diuretic therapy in preserving renal function at 96 hours (p 0.003), with no significant difference in weight loss between the two therapies and a significant increase in serious adverse events (p 0.03).

Although the results of the CARRESS-HF trial provided a strong argument against the use of ultrafiltration as primary therapy in patients with acute CRS, criticisms of the trial included the use of a different age group, and a fixed ultrafiltration rate, considered to be non-physiological, therefore further studies are needed to identify the nuances of this treatment modality (94).

Renal replacement therapy. The 2 most common modalities are peritoneal dialysis and in-center hemodialysis, with similar results according to observational studies, except for poorer survival with peritoneal dialysis (95)not yet clearly explained, probably due to inadequate fluid removal (96)Although hemodialysis three times a week in the center remains by far the most common modality, the limited duration of this regimen often necessitates more aggressive ultrafiltration, particularly in patients with chronic IC, to ensure adequate volume removal at each session and thus a large and rapid transfer of fluid considered to be an excessive stress on the heart and vascular system that is often poorly tolerated. Reduced cardiac output in patients with CHF increases the risk of perdialysis hypotension, with myocardial dysfunction, which over time becomes a major factor in the progression of CHF (97).

Hence, other HD methods, such as short daily nocturnal therapy at home, have been proposed, which are more physiological, allowing a gentler and gradual elimination of volume with a reduced risk of cardiovascular death and hospitalization; finally, further large-scale prospective studies are needed to determine the optimal approach to EER in these patients. (98).

2.   Inotropes

Inotropes, such as dopamine and milrinone, improve cardiac output and associated venous congestion, an additional property for dopamine being its dose-dependent effects on systemic and renal vascularization, at low doses it increases renal blood flow (99) In parallel, an increase in overall mortality has been described, largely due to the increased risk of arrhythmia and long-term deterioration in myocardial function. Furthermore, there is no solid evidence to support the advantages of one specific inotrope over another (63).

In the DAD-HF II trial, 161 patients with acute heart failure were randomized to either high-dose or low-dose furosemide, with or without low-dose dopamine infusion, the study showed no benefit to the addition of dopamine infusion, including no difference in urine output or worsening of renal function ; similarly, the ROSE-AHF trial, which randomized 360 patients with acute CHF and renal dysfunction to receive either low-dose dopamine or low-dose nesiritide versus placebo, showed no effect of low-dose dopamine on 72-hour urine output or renal function.
However, in subgroup analysis, there was a trend towards improved urinary response and weight loss with low-dose dopamine in patients with EF <40% (100). Although the available data do not support the routine use of intravenous inotropic agents, these drugs should still be used in patients with low cardiac output (63).

Levosimendan is a novel inotrope that binds to cardiac troponin C, sensitizing myofilaments to calcium and treatment, increasing contractility, in addition to its vasodilatory and anti-ischemic properties, hence its beneficial effect in patients with acute heart failure (101). While early small studies of levosimendan were promising, subsequent randomized trials have not shown similar success.
In the SURVIVE study, which randomized 1,327 patients with acute IC to levosimendan or dobutamine, levosimendan did not reduce all-cause mortality compared with dobutamine (102) . In the REVIVE and REVIVE II studies, despite improvements in BNP and patient self-report with levosimendan versus placebo in patients with CI, levosimendan was associated with an increased risk of adverse cardiac events and mortality (103) data on the renal effects of levosimendan in patients with CRS are limited to a few small-scale studies, of which one RCT comparing levosimendan with dobutamine in 32 patients with CI and renal failure showed that eGFR increased by 22% in the levosimendan group versus dobutamine, while the dobutamine group remained unchanged (104). Nevertheless, further large-scale prospective studies are needed to confirm levosimendan's renal effects and long-term results in SCR.
Omecamtiv mecarbil is another new inotrope that binds selectively to cardiac myosin, enhancing cardiac contractility.

In the recent randomized GALACTIC-HF trial, mecarbil omecamtiv produced a modest but statistically significant reduction in the composite event of CI or cardiovascular death versus placebo among patients with HFrEF (37% vs. 39.1%, P = 0.03). However, when the primary composite outcome was stratified into pre-specified subgroups, the benefit of omecamtiv mecarbil was not observed in patients with eGFR <60 vs. >60 ml/min per 1.73 m2. Although this is a hypothesis, further studies are needed to confirm this finding and the efficacy of omecamtiv mecarbil or other novel myotropes in patients with CRS (105).

3.   Neurohormonal modulation

Vasopressin is a neuropeptide released by the posthypophysis in response to increased plasma osmolality and decreased effective circulating volume. Elevations of vasopressin are proportional to the severity of CI and contribute to and aggravate fluid retention and congestion. (106).

Tolvaptan, a selective V2 receptor antagonist, induces electrolyte-free water loss (aquaresis) and has been considered a potentially beneficial adjunctive therapy for patients with CHF; although several trials (EVEREST, TACTICS-HF, SECRET of CHF) have demonstrated that tolvaptan results in greater weight reduction in patients with CHF, but does not reduce mortality or hospitalization for CHF, so its use remains limited (107).

4.   RAAS inhibition

IEC and ARB.
RAAS inhibition is an established treatment for heart failure patients with reduced EF and is a class I recommendation based on numerous randomized clinical trials demonstrating its improvement in morbidity and mortality (63).

Similarly, RAAS inhibition has been shown to be a cornerstone of the management of patients with CKD, slowing its progression, but there are few long-term data in the setting of CI (108)many RCTs establishing the benefits of RAAS inhibition in HFrEF have excluded patients with severe baseline renal dysfunction because of concerns about adverse effects such as worsening renal function, hyperkalemia and hypotension. Despite these limitations, observational data and post hoc analyses of existing RCTs have suggested that the benefits of

ACEIs and ARBs extend to patients with any degree of renal impairment, and that they are considered beneficial in chronic CRS, although further randomized studies are still needed for better evaluation in these patients (109).

A rise in serum creatinine may be seen following the introduction of ACE inhibitors or ARB IIs, as demonstrated in the CONSENSUS trial, where up to 11% of subjects taking enlapril experienced an initial doubling of serum creatinine; in the SOLVD trial, too, the enalapril group experienced an increase in serum creatinine of 0.1 mg/dl on average, and 10.7% of patients experienced an increase in serum creatinine greater than 2mg/dL.

However, increases in serum creatinine tend to occur early in the course of treatment initiation, returning to less than 30% of baseline in most patients. Despite the increased rate of AKI with ACEIs, discontinuation of the drug is rarely necessary, as shown by a meta-analysis by Flather et al; when hyperkalemia occurs with the use of an ACEI or ARB II, potassium chelators may be a strategy to minimize the risk and continue treatment. Thus, the use of ACE inhibitors and ARBs, even in advanced stages of CKD, is reasonable provided that renal function and potassium levels are carefully monitored (110).

Angiotensin-neprilysin receptor blocker The combination of valsartan with sacubitril, a neprilysin inhibitor, appears to provide additional benefit over RAAS blockade alone, due in part to the additional vasodilatory effect induced by increased natriuretic peptide levels. In sub-analyses of the PARADIGM-HF and PARAGON-HF trials, the angiotensin-neprilysin receptor blocker was associated with a slowing of the decline in eGFR, and the development of ESRD in patients with CHF. Recently, the HARP-III trial, which randomized CKD patients between ARNI and irbesartan, showed no additional renal benefit of ARNI over RAAS blockade.

In the HARP-III study, cardiac biomarkers troponin I and NT-proBNP were significantly reduced in the ARNI group, leading the investigators to hypothesize a probable reduction in cardiovascular risk in CKD patients on ARNI, but further studies as to its safety and efficacy in CKD are required, since so far a small prospective study by Lee and his team reported improved LVEF in HFrEF patients on dialysis with ARNI with dose reduction, without stopping treatment in 21% of patients at follow-up due to adverse effects (111,112).

Mineralocorticoid receptor antagonist (MRA)

Additional inhibition of the RAAS system by a mineralocorticoid antagonist offers long-term cardiovascular benefits for heart failure patients, as demonstrated by the RALES, EPHESUS and especially EMPHASIS-HF trials, which showed a clear improvement in cardiovascular morbidity and mortality in patients with moderate CKD (63) ; on the other hand, the EPHESUS study also highlighted the cardiovascular benefits of eplerenone, despite the acute deterioration in GFR observed following its introduction; it should be noted that this molecule did not influence the slope of the decline in GFR in the trial. However, finerenone, a selective non-steroidal MRA, is a new molecule with a proven track record in reducing the rate of progression of CKD and cardiovascular events in patients with CKD and type II diabetes (113) but data in patients with heart failure or advanced CKD remain limited, and current CI guidelines indicate spironolactone for patients with a GFR >30 ml/min per 1.73 m^2.

5.   Beta-blockers

While the benefits of beta-blockers are well established in CI on the basis of large-scale RCTs, data in CKD remain limited to observational studies or post hoc analyses of RCTs.

The MERIT-HF study, which assessed the effects of metoprolol at different eGFR values, concluded that patients with the lowest eGFR (<45 ml/min per 1.73 m2) benefited most from the drug, with a greater reduction in the risk of cardiovascular events in this proportion of patients, and a nearly 60% reduction in mortality and hospitalization for heart failure. (114). Similarly, a randomized trial of 114 dialysis patients followed for CMD showed superiority of carvedilol over placebo on lower mortality (115). On the other hand, a meta-analysis of the CAPRICORN and COPERNICIC studies showed that carvedilol showed a benefit in acute IC with eGFR >45ml/min/1.73m² only (116). A subsequent meta-analysis of 10 RCTs including 16,740 patients with LVEF <50% showed a clear reduction in mortality by beta-blockers in mild to moderate CKD with limited data in severe CKD due to the small sample of patients in this proportion, and some caution regarding the tolerability of beta-blockers due to the specificities of this population (fluid retention, bradycardia and hypotension) (117) .

6.   SGLT2 inhibitors (SGLT2i)

In addition to their ability to reduce major adverse cardiac events in diabetics with established CVD or at high risk of CVD(63) , current trials are looking at the effects of SGLT2i in patients with CI, We cite the DAPA-HF and EMPEROR-Reduced trials, both of which showed a significant reduction in cardiovascular death or hospitalization for CHF with the use of SGLT2i versus placebo, irrespective of the presence of diabetes, in addition to a notable renoprotective effect.

Although their mechanism of action has yet to be fully elucidated, the glycosuric and natriuretic effect is responsible for lowering intra-glomerular hydrostatic pressures, and has a protective effect on glomerular function, (On the other hand, it significantly reduces cardiac filling pressures, making it easier to manage congestion in patients with chronic heart failure. As the site of inhibition of sodium reabsorption with SGLT2i is close to the macula densa, there is little compensatory neurohormonal activation with these molecules, hence their long-term cardio-renal benefits (118,119).

7.   Device-based therapy

Implantable cardioverter defibrillators. The MADIT, MUSTT and SCD-HeFT trials, among others, have clearly demonstrated the advantage of ICDs in terms of mortality in IC patients, particularly those with ischemic cardiomyopathy, whereas their value in moderate CKD is less clear. (120)especially when the cohort of Bansal et al. including 5877 heart failure patients with CKD, showed an association with an increased risk of subsequent hospitalization for CI and all causes, and with the risk of sudden cardiac death, but deaths due to concurrent non-cardiac causes are also high in this population, thus attenuating the benefits of ICD therapy, which is why the decision to implant must take into account the patient's frailty and quality of life when assessing the risk for these patients (121).

Recently, subcutaneous ICDs have been developed with comparable efficacy to transvenous ICDs, as demonstrated by the recent UNTOUCHED trial in which the use of an S-ICD was associated with almost 96% freedom from inappropriate shocks at 18 months, which is similar to the data on transvenous ICDs but with fewer complications; they are moreover preferable in patients with advanced

CKD or ESRD with vascular access problems; finally, further studies are still needed (122).

Cardiac resynchronization therapy. Cardiac resynchronization therapy (CRT) in medically refractory heart failure patients reduced all-cause mortality and improved symptoms by improving ejection fraction through synchronous biventricular pacing irrespective of eGFR, with significant increases in eGFR and decreases in uremia in patients with moderate CKD as demonstrated by the MIRACLE study including 453 patients with NYHA class III-IV CHF, with LVEF <35% and QRS >130 ms. Despite these advantages, overall mortality in patients with concomitant CHF and CKD remains high, and further studies are needed to determine which patients with CKD are likely to benefit most from this therapy (123).

8.   Mechanical circulatory support

Mechanical circulatory support devices are used as an option for patients with advanced heart failure or as a bridge to heart transplantation, where there is often an early increase in eGFR due to improved flow and hemodynamics, as demonstrated by the retrospective study by Hasin et al where 67% of patients with moderate to severe CKD who underwent implantation of a continuous-flow LVAD (HeartMate II), improved to an eGFR >60 ml/min/1.73 m2 at 1 month (124) but these changes tended to regress over time, approaching pre-implantation eGFR levels at 12 months (125) partly due to chronic activation of the RAAS with reduced pulsatile flow and smooth muscle hypertrophy in the renal cortical arteries secondary to continuous flow, which will impair renal function; on the other hand, determining the reversibility of renal dysfunction prior to sustained LVAD implantation is often difficult to predict: ancillary studies suggesting irreversible CKD include renal imaging identifying small kidneys or persistent proteinuria >0.5 g/d, renal biopsy may also be useful to identify the extent of tubular atrophy/interstitial fibrosis in order to quantify the extent of irreversible renal failure, but these are difficult to perform, particularly in this critically ill population (126,127).

9.   Heart and kidney transplants

Renal transplantation. Renal transplantation for patients with end-stage renal disease is associated with better quality of life and cost-effectiveness for the healthcare system compared with dialysis (128) but the presence of heart failure is associated with poorer outcomes, with an estimated 2.5% mortality while awaiting transplantation (129) once transplanted, patients with reduced LVEF have higher rates of delayed recovery of graft function and longer renal recovery times before being dialysis-free (130).

Particular attention is paid to people with "uremic cardiomyopathy" prior to transplantation, in whom transplantation improves LVEF, highlighting the relationship between CI and CKD (8).

Heart transplantation. This is an effective treatment option for patients with end-stage heart failure; studies of heart transplant patients show that pre-transplant eGFR is independently associated with post-transplant mortality and ESRD (131)renal function following cardiac transplantation is generally considered to follow a progressive decline, as demonstrated by a study of 151 transplant patients followed over 9 years, in which an average 44% fall in eGFR was observed, almost 10 times the rate expected in the general population; this decline is probably multifactorial and linked to treatment with calcineurin inhibitors, the effects of hypertension and hypercholesterolemia, repeated coronary angiography and possible immune-mediated effects (132).

Combined heart and kidney transplantation is an option for heart transplant patients with severe baseline renal failure, supported by data from the United Network for Organ Sharing (UNOS) registry (133) which suggest that combined transplantation overcomes the survival disadvantage associated with preoperative renal dysfunction observed with heart transplantation alone and may be a preferable option in these patients.

Another option is renal transplantation after cardiac transplantation in patients who develop ESRD following cardiac transplantation (133,134)but it is often difficult to differentiate between patients in whom renal failure is due to a reversible cause versus intrinsic renal disease, and clinical practice varies considerably; this distinction is essential because in patients with presumed CRS, restoration of cardiac output in the acute setting will often result in improved renal function, whereas in patients with intrinsic renal disease, such renal recovery is not expected; current consensus guidelines recommend considering simultaneous cardio-renal transplantation in heart transplant candidates with established moderate-to-severe CKD (small kidneys on imaging, persistent proteinuria >0.5g/day), although further studies are needed to define optimal patient selection criteria (112).

10. Palliative care

Advanced CRS is synonymous with poor prognosis and quality of life. In addition to the physical symptoms of CHF, depression is also prevalent in this population, but remains underdiagnosed and undertreated despite being an independent predictor of mortality and worsening of CHF symptoms in patients with advanced CRS, highlighting the potential benefits of palliative care in this patient population, as demonstrated by a meta-analysis of 15 studies suggesting that these interventions induce improved outcomes with a reduction in the risk of rehospitalization of up to 44% (135,136).

VIII. ILLUSTRIOUS CLINICAL CASES

Clinical case n° 1

Patient D.M., aged 59, married, tradesman by profession, from Algiers, history of NIDDM, hypertension, followed for dilated cardiomyopathy since 2017, treated with Carvedilol 6.25 mg/d, furosemide 40 in four doses per day and Ramipril 2.5 mg /d, under oral anticoagulation with antivitamin K (Acenocoumarol) admitted to the cardiology department for global cardiac decompensation predominantly right.

On admission

The patient was in average general condition, dyspneic with bilateral lower limb edema (OMI), blood pressure 110/80 mm Hg, SpO2 94%, heart rate 92 bpm. Weight was 96 kg for a height of 1.80 m. Clinical examination revealed cervical adenopathy with hepatomegaly but no splenomegaly.

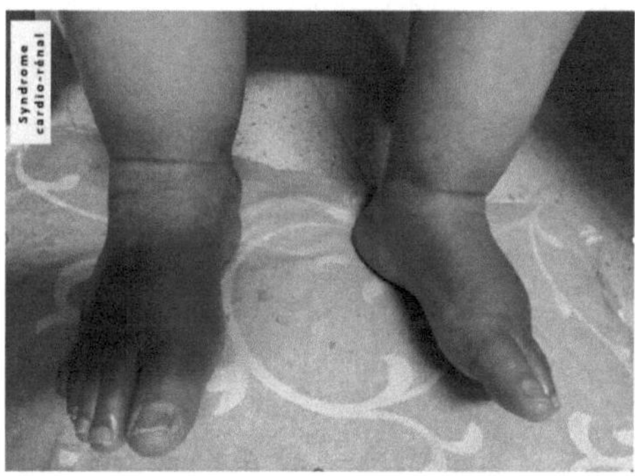

Figure 1: Edema of the lower limbs

The ECG showed atrial fibrillation at 84 bpm, with planing of the R waves anteriorly, with respect for the QRS inferiorly.

Biological tests showed anemia with hemoglobin at 9.7 g/dl, platelets at 166,000/mm^3 and leukocytes at 3000/mm^3· Renal function was impaired with urea at 0.62 g/l and creatinine at 20 mg/l. CRP was 5.3 mg/l, natremia 137 meq/l and kalemia 3.7 meq/l.

What to do

In an emergency, condition the patient, start treatment with an IV loop diuretic: Furosemide 60 mg 3x/d and maintain anticoagulation with Acenocoumarol with a target INR.

Cervical ultrasound on 11/05/2023 revealed supraclavicular adenopathy. Abdominal and pelvic ultrasound on 08/05/2023 revealed congestive hepatomegaly with portal hypertension syndrome and large ascites secondary to cardiac disease, cardiomegaly with pulmonary interstitial syndrome suggestive of acute pulmonary edema.

Doppler echocardiography on 12/11/2021 showed dilated heart disease with left ventricular systolic and diastolic dysfunction, dilated right heart chambers, PAH, free pericardium, EF: 35%, grade 3 MI, dilated OG, global hypokinesia, grade 2 IT.

Given the increase in edema, ascites and low diuresis on diuretics, ultrafiltration sessions were indicated.

Start of sessions on 14/05/2023, every other day, with depletion of 2 to 3 kg/session

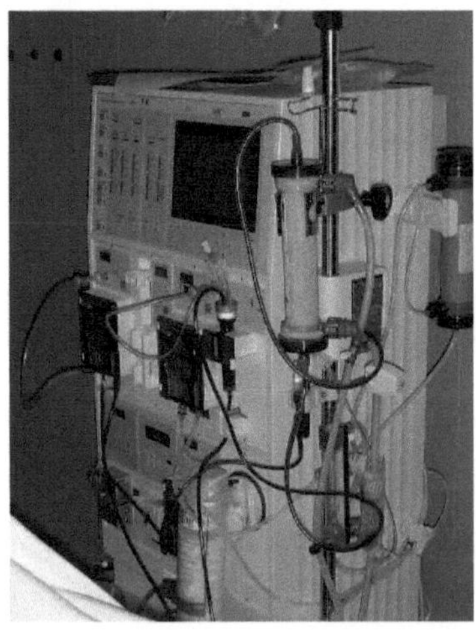

Figure 2: Fresenius 4008 dialysis machine

The assessment on 21/05/2023 showed an NSF with WBC at 4950/mm^3 , Hb at 8.8, Hte at 27.8%, VGM at 88.8 fl, CCMH at 31.5 and platelets at 220 G/mm$^{3.}$

After six ultrafiltration sessions, the patient was depleted, weight dropped by 12 kg, edema regressed, ascites disappeared and general condition improved.

Clinical case n°2

Patient H.Y. born in 1950, aged 73, admitted on 6/12/2022 to the Cardiology Department for recurrent cardiac decompensation.

In his history, the patient has several cardiovascular risk factors, arterial hypertension on treatment, type 2 diabetes on insulin, abdominal obesity, obstructive sleep apnea and hypopnea syndrome (OSAHS), unknown chronic renal failure; he was implanted with a pace maker in VVI mode in March 2022 following an atrioventricular block on complete arrhythmia by permanent atrial fibrillation. He is also being monitored for heart failure.

The history of the disease

The patient had been ill for several weeks, with the onset of edema of the IM and progressively worsening ascites. On admission, the patient was conscious, cooperative, dyspneic type III, apyretic, hemodynamically stable, BP 95/53 mm Hg, HR 72 bpm, SpO2 99%. Weight 88 kg and height 174 cm.

Examination revealed signs of right heart failure: IMO, abundant ascites and turgidity of peripheral veins.

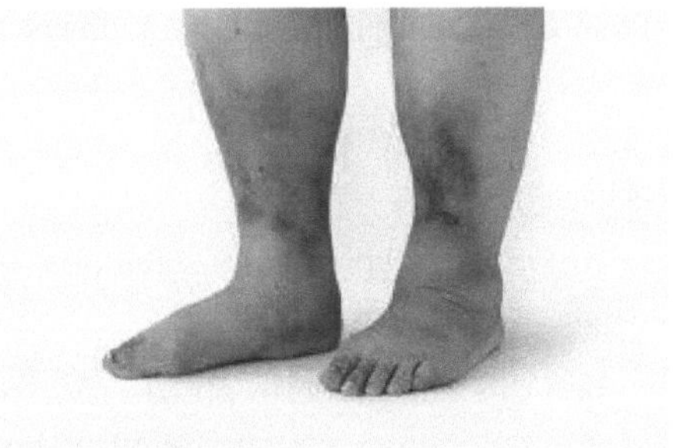

Figure 3: Edema of the lower limbs

Cardiac auscultation revealed well-struck heart sounds, pulmonary auscultation was unobstructed, and neurological examination revealed a conscious patient with a score of 15/15.

The ECG showed an electrostimulated rhythm at 72 bpm. Biological tests showed renal failure with urea at 2.93 g/l, creatinine at 23 mg/l and GFR at 29 ml/min/1.73 m^2. Natremia was 134 meq/l and potassium 3.7 meq/l, AST 31 IU/l, ALT 20 IU/l,

PAL 81 IU/l, albumin 39 g/l, BT 14 mg/l and BD 9 mg/l. FNS showed WBC 6330/µl, Hb 8.8 g/dl and platelets 232,000/mm^3 . INR was 1.38.

<u>Intra-hospital treatment</u> consisted of conditioning, starting Furosemide at SAP at 3cc/h, hydrochlorothiazide: 25 mg/d, Spironolactone: 75 mg ½ cp /d and scheduling hemodialysis sessions with transfusion of packed red blood cells.

Abdominal and renal ultrasound revealed hyperechoic kidneys with loss of cortico-medullary differentiation.

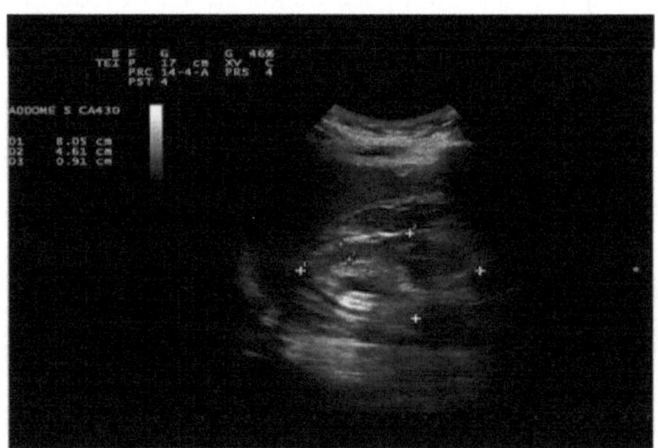

Figure 4: Abdominal-renal ultrasound: hyperechoic kidneys

<u>Development in the department</u>

The patient was conscious, in BEG, hemodynamically stable, BP 140/70 mmHg, HR 60 bpm, SpO2 99%, no signs of ICD or ICG.

Cardiac echocardiography: non-dilated, hypertrophied LV, preserved EF, presence of kinetic disturbances at the septum, elevated PDR, PH of intermediate probability, dry pericardium, basally dilated LV with borderline systolic function.

 Biological tests revealed urea at 1.42 g/l, creatinine at 23 mg/l, Natremia at 136 meq/l, Kalemia at 3.9 meq/l, AST at 31 IU/l, ALT at 20 IU/l, PAL at 81 IU/l, albumin at 39 g/l, BT at 17 mg/l.

FNS objectified WBC at 5340/µl (L at 0.85_x10 /mm^{33} , PNN at 3.7_x10 /mm^{33} , PNE at 0.17_x10 /mm^{33} , MN at 0.5_x10 /mm^{33}), Hb at 8.7 g/dl, Hte at 27.6%, VGM at 90.7 fl, CCMH at 31.7, platelets at 247,000/mm^3.

On day 23 of hospitalization, the patient was hemodynamically stable, diuresis 4.5 l/24h, renal function still impaired with urea 2 g/l, creatinine 21 mg/l, Natremia 135 and hypokalemia 2.8 meq/l. INR 1.85.

Our course of action was to lower the furosemide, switch to IV bolus 60 mg 3_x/d and give a potassium load to SAP (1gr in 60 cc to be renewed 4X/d).

At d25, diuresis was 4000 cc/24H, prompting discontinuation of IV furosemide.

<u>TRT at the exit:</u>

The patient was discharged on oral therapy with Furosemide 500 mg/d, Aldactone 75 mg/l ½ cp /d and sintrom 1/4 cp/d with referral letter to Nephrology.

<u>The patient was readmitted to hospital</u> on 04/05/2023 for right heart decompensation.

The history goes back 5 days, marked by the appearance of edema of the lower limbs.

Clinical <u>examination</u> revealed a patient in moderate EG, with significant IMO, abundant ascites and preserved diuresis: signs of right and left heart failure, HR at 84 bpm, BP at 130/107 mmHg.

Blood tests showed urea at 2.78 g/l, creatinine at 29 mg/l, Natremia at 129 meq/l and Kalemia at 4.6 meq/l.

During hospitalization, renal failure worsened, with urea at 2.98 g/l, creatinine at 30 mg/l, and oliguria with diuresis at 0.5 l/d.

<u>What to do</u>

Furosemide 3cc/H reintroduced at SAP and Ultrafiltration sessions indicated. On 10/5/2023, with urea at 2.88 and creatinine at 32 mg/l, HD was started with transfusion of a packed red blood cell (RBC).

On 5/14/2023, urea increased to 3 g/l, creatinine to 40 mg/l, and hyponatremia set in at 125 meq/l, prompting intensification of ultrafiltration sessions.

<u>Evolution</u>

During hospitalization, the patient presented with fever and hyperleukocytosis. Blood cultures revealed a group KES enterobacter sensitive to cefotaxime and ciprofloxacin. UF was continued with CG transfusion.

<u>Cardiac Doppler ultrasound</u>

A non-dilated, hypertrophied LV with preserved systolic function and EF: 58%. Moderate to moderate tricuspid leak, high filling pressures, dilated right cavities, LV with borderline systolic function. PH of intermediate probability, dry pericardium.

CAT: continue UF sessions every 48 hours with dialysis (UF 2l /session)

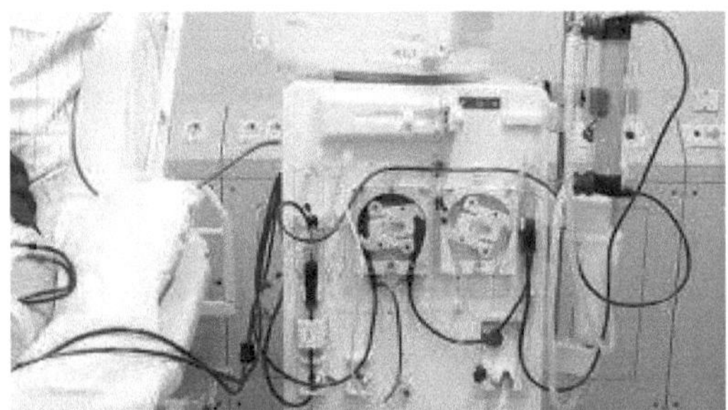

Figure 5: Ultrafiltration with a hemodialysis machine

After 10 haemodialysis sessions, clinical condition improved, patient lost 13 kg, oedema disappeared, urea and creatinine levels fell to 1 g/l and 20 mg/l respectively.

Clinical case 3

Patient R.B., age 71, admitted on 05/15/2023 for infective endocarditis of native mitral valve complicated by severe MI in heart failure (PAO and ICG).

The patient's history includes type 2 diabetes on insulin, arterial hypertension and benign prostatic hypertrophy.

<u>History of the disease</u>

Two weeks ago, in the face of the onset of an infectious syndrome, a telethorax performed on 8/5/2023 revealed a basal right parenchymal opacity with a watery tone, heterogeneous area, poorly limited (probable focus of infectious pneumopathy), and the diagnosis of pneumopathy was made.

A week later, he had an emergency cardiology consultation for PAO and suspected infective endocarditis.

Examination revealed a patient with altered general condition, orthopnea, MI murmur 4/6, 2/3 crepitus rales, IMO and BP 110/70 mmHg. Neurologically, the patient was drowsy, scored 15/15.

Arterial network: pulses present throughout, no signs of pseudoaneurysm or arteriovenous fistula. Venous network: no signs of deep vein thrombosis.

The search for an entry point revealed poor oral hygiene and intertrigo.

A telethorax revealed bilateral interstitial oedema.

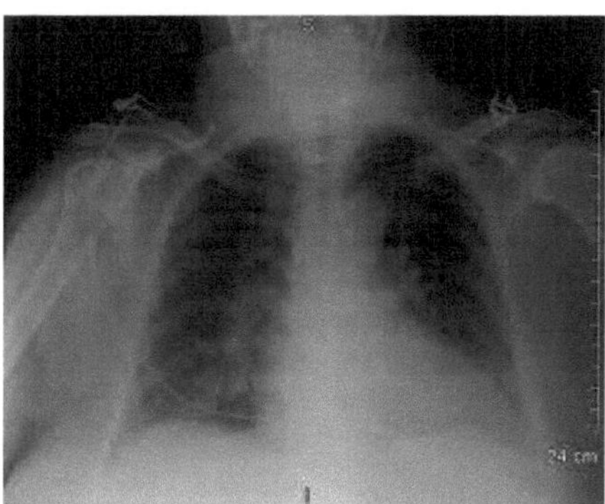

Figure 6: Bilateral interstitial edema (OAP)

Emergency echocardiography had revealed an anechoic mass on the ventricular face of the large mitral valve suggestive of mutilating vegetation (20X15 mm), massive MI due to A2 prolapse on probable cord rupture, a non-hypertrophied LV of borderline size with good systolic function and 60% EF, a dilated OG, a non-dilated VD with good function, TAPS at 24mm, significant IT, high probability PH (PAPS at 70 mm) and dry pericardium.

Biological tests on 13/5/2023 showed blood glucose at 2.43 g/l, urea at 2.89 g/l, creatinine at 29 mg/l, CRP at 102 mg/l, Natremia at 118 meq/l and Kalemia at 5 meq/l.

FNS showed Hb 8.7 g/dl, Hte 27.7%, VGM 79.9 fl, CCMH 31.3, WBC 20340/mm^3 , PNN 89.9%, platelets 503000/mm^3 and PT 81%.

The ECG showed a regular sinus rhythm, fine QRS and no repolarization disorders.

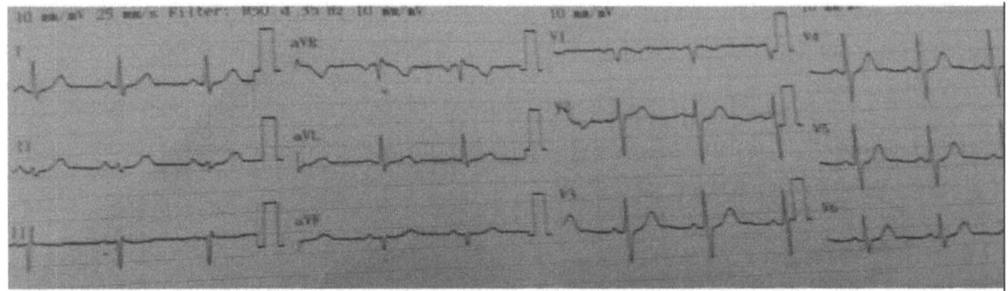

Figure 7: ECG showing fine QRS, no repolarization disorders

What to do

Hydro-sodium restriction was instituted, with urine quantification and urine ionogram, and blood cultures were taken.

Dialysis was started on 18/05/2023 with injection of vancomycin 1g/10 d and gentamycin 1mg/kg/d for 3 d.

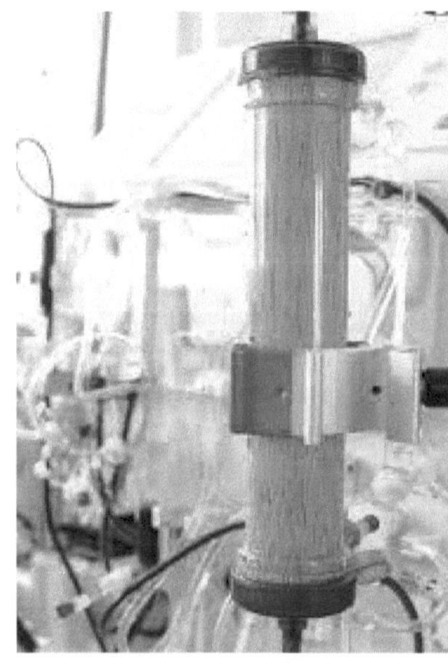

May 20: signs of left ventricular failure, BP 110/70 mm Hg, crepitus in the lower 1/3.

On 05/21, an ultrafiltration session was performed. Results showed urea at 1.67 g/l and creatinine at 16 mg/l.

Hemodialysis sessions were stopped on 22/05 after improvement in renal function and disappearance of signs of PAO.

Bibliography

1. Ronco C, McCullough P, Anker SD, et al. Cardio-renal syndromes: report from the consensus conference of the acute dialysis quality initiative. Eur Heart J 2010;31:703-11.

2. House AA, Anand I, Bellomo R, et al. Definition and classification of cardio-renal syndromes: work_group statements from the 7th ADQI consensus conference. Nephrol Dial Transplant 2010;25(5): 1416-20.

3. Ronco C, House AA, Haapio M. Cardiorenal syndrome: refining the definition of a complex symbiosis gone wrong. Intensive Care Med 2008; 34(5):957.

4. Health, United States. With special feature on mortality, 87, 2017. Available at: https://www.cdc. gov/nchs/data/hus/hus17.pdf.

5. Damman K, Tang WHW, Testani JM, et al. Terminology and definition of changes renal function in heart failure. Eur Heart J 2014;35(48):3413-6.

6. Bagshaw SM, Cruz DN, Aspromonte N, et al. Epidemiology of cardio-renal syn_dromes: workgroup statements from the 7th ADQI Consensus Conference. Nephrol Dial Transplant 2010;25:1406-16.

7. Cheung AK, Sarnak MJ, Yan G, et al. Cardiac diseases in maintenance hemodialysis patients: results of the HEMO Study. Kidney Int 2004;65:2380-9.

8. Rangaswami J, Bhalla V, Blair JE, et al. Cardiorenal syndrome: classification, path_ophysiology, diagnosis, and treatment strategies: a scientific statement from the American Heart Association. Circulation 2019;139:e840-e78.

9. Vallabhajosyula S, Sakhuja A, Geske JB, et al. Clinical profile and outcomes of acute cardiorenal syndrome type-5 in sepsis: An eight-year cohort study. PLoS One 2018;13:e0190965.

10. Almaani S, Meara A, Rovin BH. Update on lupus nephritis. Clin J Am Soc Nephrol 2017;12:825-35.

11.   Rezk T, Lachmann HJ, Fontana M, et al. Cardiorenal AL amyloidosis: risk stratifica_tion and outcomes based upon cardiac and renal biomarkers. Br J Haematol 2019;186:460-70.

12.   Lu JY, Buczek A, Fleysher R, et al. Outcomes of hospitalized patients with COVID_19 with acute kidney injury and acute cardiac injury. Front Cardiovasc Med 2021;8:798897.

13.   Khwaja A. KDIGO clinical practice guidelines for acute kidney injury. Nephron Clin Pract 2012; 120(4):c179-84.

14.   Malbrain ML, Cheatham ML, Kirkpatrick A, et al. Results from the international conference of experts on intra-abdominal hypertension and abdominal compartment syndrome. I. Definitions. Intensive Care Med 2006;32(11):1722-32.

15.   Dalfino L, Tullo L, Donadio I, et al. Intra-abdominal hypertension and acute renal failure in critically ill patients. Intensive Care Med 2008;34(4):707-13.

16.   Mullens W, Abrahams Z, Skouri HN, et al. Elevated intra-abdominal pressure in acute decompensated heart failure: a potential contributor to worsening renal function? J Am Coll Cardiol 2008;51(3): 300-6.

17.   Damman K, van Deursen VM, Navis G, et al. Increased central venous pressure is associated with impaired renal function and mortality in a broad spectrum of patients with cardiovascular disease. J Am Coll Cardiol 2009;53(7):582-8.

18.   Maeder MT, Holst DP, Kaye DM. Tricuspid regurgi_tation contributes to renal dysfunction in patients with heart failure. J Card Fail 2008;14(10):824-30.

19.   Binanay C, Califf RM, Hasselblad V, et al. Evalua_tion study of congestive heart failure and pulmo_nary artery catheterization effectiveness: the ESCAPE trial. JAMA 2005;294(13):1625-33.

20.   Tarvasma¨ki T, Haapio M, Mebazaa A, et al. Acute kidney injury in cardiogenic shock: definitions, inci_dence, haemodynamic alterations, and mortality. Eur J Heart Fail 2018;20(3):572-81.

21.   Lauschke A, Teichgra¨ber UKM, Frei U, et al. 'Low_dose' dopamine worsens renal perfusion in pa_tients with acute renal failure. Kidney Int 2006; 69(9):1669-74.

22.   Ferrario CM, Strawn WB. Role of the renin_angiotensin-aldosterone system and proinflamma_tory mediators in cardiovascular disease. Am J Cardiol 2006;98(1):121-8.

23.   Kopp UC. Neural control of renin secretion rate. Morgan & Claypool Life Sciences; 2011. Available at: https://www.ncbi.nlm.nih.gov/books/NBK57240/. Accessed January 3, 2019.

24.   Harrison-Bernard LM. The renal renin-angiotensin system. Adv Physiol Educ 2009;33(4):270-4.

25.   Barton M, Shaw S, d'uscio LV, et al. Angiotensin II increases vascular and renal endothelin-1 and functional endothelin converting enzyme activity in vivo: role of ETA receptors for endothelin regula_tion. Biochem Biophys Res Commun 1997;238(3): 861-5.

26   Hitomi H, Kiyomoto H, Nishiyama A. Angiotensin II and oxidative stress. Curr Opin Cardiol 2007;22(4): 311-5.

27.   Funaya H, Kitakaze M, Node K, et al. Plasma aden_osine levels increase in patients with chronic heart failure. Circulation 1997;95(6):1363-5.

28.   Massie BM, O'Connor CM, Metra M, et al. Rolofyl_line, an adenosine A1_Receptor antagonist, in acute heart failure. N Engl J Med 2010;363(15): 1419-28.

29.   Torres VE. Vasopressin in chronic kidney disease, an elephant in the room? Kidney Int 2009;76(9): 925-8.

30.   Rubattu S, Mennuni S, Testa M, et al. Pathogenesis of chronic cardiorenal syndrome: is there a role for oxidative stress? Int J Mol Sci 2013;14(11): 23011-32.

31.   Virzi` GM, Clementi A, de Cal M, et al. Oxidative stress: dual pathway induction in cardiorenal syn_drome type 1 pathogenesis. Oxid Med Cell Longev 2015;2015. https://doi.org/10.1155/2015/391790.

32.   Chabrashvili T, Kitiyakara C, Blau J, et al. Effects of ANG II type 1 and 2 receptors on oxidative stress, renal NADPH oxidase, and SOD expression. Am J Physiol Regul Integr Comp Physiol 2003;285(1): R117-24.

33.   Ushio-Fukai M, Zafari AM, Fukui T, et al. P22phox is a critical component of the superoxide-generating NADH/NADPH oxidase system and regulates angiotensin II-induced hypertrophy in vascular smooth muscle cells. J Biol Chem 1996;271(38): 23317-21.

34.   Modaresi A, Nafar M, Sahraei Z. Oxidative stress in chronic kidney disease 2015;9(3):15.

35.   Wettersten N, Maisel AS. Biomarkers for heart fail_ure: an update for practitioners of internal medi_cine. Am J Med 2016;129(6):560-7.

36.   Stenvinkel P, Ketteler M, Johnson RJ, et al. IL-10, IL-6, and TNF-alpha: central factors in the altered cytokine network of uremia-the good, the bad, and the ugly. Kidney Int 2005;67(4):1216-33.

37.   Cermak J, Key NS, Bach RR, et al. C-reactive protein induces human peripheral blood mono_cytes to synthesize tissue factor. Blood 1993;82(2): 513-20. Available at: http://www.bloodjournal.org/ content/82/2/513. Accessed January 22, 2019.

38.   Minami Y, Kajimoto K, Sato N, et al. Effect of elevated C-reactive protein level at discharge on long-term outcome in patients hospitalized for acute heart failure. Am J Cardiol 2018;121(8):961-8.

39.   Kim B-S, Jeon DS, Shin MJ, et al. Persistent eleva_tion of C-reactive protein may predict cardiac hy_pertrophy and dysfunction in patients maintained on hemodialysis. Am J Nephrol 2005;25(3):189-95.

40.   Chinnappa S, Tu Y-K, Yeh YC, et al. Association between protein-bound uremic toxins and asymp_tomatic cardiac dysfunction in patients with chronic kidney disease. Toxins (Basel) 2018; 10(12). https://doi.org/10.3390/toxins10120520.

41.   Lin C-J, Liu H-L, Pan C-F, et al. Indoxyl sulfate pre_dicts cardiovascular disease and renal function deterioration in advanced chronic kidney disease. Arch Med Res 2012;43(6):451-6.

42.   Wu I-W, Hsu K-H, Lee C-C, et al. p-Cresyl sulphate and indoxyl sulphate predict progression of chronic kidney disease. Nephrol Dial Transplant 2011;26(3):938-47.

43.   Barreto FC, Barreto DV, Liabeuf S, et al. Serum indoxyl sulfate is associated with vascular disease and mortality in chronic kidney disease patients. Clin J Am Soc Nephrol 2009;4(10):1551-8.

44.   Kao Y-H, Chen Y-C, Lin Y-K, et al. FGF-23 dysregu_lates calcium homeostasis and electrophysiolog_ical properties in HL-1 atrial cells. Eur J Clin Invest 2014;44(8):795-801.

45.   Adams KF, Patterson JH, Oren RM, et al. Prospec_tive assessment of the occurrence of anemia in pa_tients with heart failure: results from the study of anemia in a heart failure population (STAMINA_HFP) registry. Am Heart J 2009;157(5):

46.   Young JB, Abraham WT, Albert NM, et al. Relation of low hemoglobin and anemia to morbidity and mortality in patients hospitalized with heart failure (insight from the OPTIMIZE-HF registry). Am J Car_diol 2008;101(2):223-30.

47.   McClellan W, Aronoff SL, Bolton WK, et al. The prevalence of anemia in patients with chronic kid_ney disease. Curr Med Res Opin 2004;20(9): 1501-10.

48   Grune T, Sommerburg O, Siems WG. Oxidative stress in anemia. Clin Nephrol 2000;53(1 Suppl):S18-22. Available at: http://europepmc.org/abstract/med/ 10746801. Accessed January 21, 2019.

49   Denton KM, Shweta A, Anderson WP. Pre_glomerular and postglomerular resistance re_sponses to different levels of sympathetic activation by hypoxia. J Am Soc Nephrol 2002; 13(1):27-34. Available at: https://jasn.asnjournals. org/content/13/1/27. Accessed January 21, 2019.

50.   Singh AK, Szczech L, Tang KL, et al. Correction of anemia with epoetin alfa in chronic kidney disease. N Engl J Med 2006;355(20):2085-98.

51.   Pfeffer MA, Burdmann EA, Chen C-Y, et al. A trial of darbepoetin alfa in type 2 diabetes and chronic kidney disease. N Engl J Med 2009;361(21): 2019-32.

52.   Swedberg K, Young JB, Anand IS, et al. Treatment of anemia with darbepoetin alfa in systolic heart failure. N Engl J Med 2013;368(13):1210-9.

53.   Mehta RL, Rabb H, Shaw AD, et al. Cardiorenal syndrome type 5: clinical presentation, pathophys_iology and management strategies from the elev_enth consensus conference of the Acute Dialysis Quality Initiative (ADQI). Contrib Nephrol 2013; 182:174-94.

54.   Di Lullo L, Bellasi A, Barbera V, et al. Pathophysi_ology of the cardio-renal syndromes types 1-5: an uptodate. Indian Heart J 2017;69(2):255-65.

55.   Hatamizadeh P, Fonarow GC, Budoff MJ, et al. Car_diorenal syndrome: pathophysiology and potential targets for clinical management. Nat Rev Nephrol 2013;9(2):99-111.

56.   van Kimmenade RR, Januzzi JL, Jr, Baggish AL, et al. Amino-terminal pro-brain natriuretic Peptide, renal function, and outcomes in acute heart failure: redefining the cardiorenal interaction? J Am Coll Cardiol 2006;48:1621-7.

57.   McCallum W, Tighiouart H, Kiernan MS, Huggins GS, Sarnak MJ. Relation of kid_ney function decline and NT-proBNP with risk of mortality and readmission in acute decompensated heart failure. Am J Med 2020;133:115-22. e2.

58.   Wu AH, Wians F, Jaffe A. Biological variation of galectin-3 and soluble ST2 for chronic heart failure: implication on interpretation of test results. Am Heart J 2013;165:995-9.

59.   Ng LL, Squire IB, Jones DJL, et al. Proenkephalin, renal dysfunction, and prognosis in patients with acute heart failure: a great network study. J Am Coll Cardiol 2017;69:56-69.

60.   Lena A, Anker MS, Springer J. Muscle wasting and sarcopenia in heart failure-the current state of science. Int J Mol Sci 2020;21:6549.

61   Lassus J, Harjola VP. Cystatin C: a step forward in assessing kidney function and cardiovascular risk. Heart Fail Rev 2012;17:251-61.

62.   Roos JF, Doust J, Tett SE, Kirkpatrick CM. Diagnostic accuracy of cystatin C com_pared to serum creatinine for the estimation of renal dysfunction in adults and child_ren_a meta-analysis. Clin Biochem 2007;40:383-91.

63.   Jackson CE, Solomon SD, Gerstein HC, et al. Albuminuria in chronic heart failure: prevalence and prognostic importance. Lancet (London, England) 2009;374:543- 50.

64.   Mi~nana G, Ll_acer P, Sanchis I, et al. Early spot urinary sodium and diuretic effi_ciency in acute heart failure and concomitant renal dysfunction. Cardiorenal Med 2020;10:362-72.

65.   Mavrakanas TA, Khattak A, Singh K, Charytan DM. Epidemiology and natural his_tory of the cardiorenal syndromes in a cohort with echocardiography. Clin J Am Soc Nephrol 2017;12:1624-33.

66.   Tandon R, Mohan B, ST Chhabra, Aslam N, Wander GS. Clinical and echocardio_graphic predictors of cardiorenal syndrome type I in patients with acute ischemic right ventricular dysfunction. Cardiorenal Med 2013;3:239-45.

67.   Heidenreich PA, Bozkurt B, Aguilar D, et al. 2022 AHA/ACC/HFSA guideline for the management of heart failure: a report of the American college of cardiology/American heart association joint committee on clinical practice guidelines. J Am Coll Cardiol 2022;79:e263-421.

68.   Hassanin N, Alkemary A. Early detection of subclinical uremic cardiomyopathy using two-dimensional speckle tracking echocardiography. Echocardiography 2016;33:527–36.

69.   Iida N, Seo Y, Sai S, et al. Clinical implications of intrarenal hemodynamic evalua_tion by doppler ultrasonography in heart failure. JACC Heart Fail 2016;4:674-82.

70.   Rutherford E, Talle MA, Mangion K, et al. Defining myocardial tissue abnormalities in end-stage renal failure with cardiac magnetic resonance imaging using native T1 mapping. Kidney Int 2016;90:845-52.

71. Breidthardt T, Cox EF, Squire I, et al. The pathophysiology of the chronic cardiore_nal syndrome: a magnetic resonance imaging study. Eur Rad.

72. Eisenberg PR, Jaffe AS, Schuster DP. Clinical evaluation compared to pulmonary artery catheterization in the hemodynamic assessment of critically ill patients. Crit Care Med 1984;12:549-53.

73. Grodin JL, Drazner MH, Dupont M, et al. A disproportionate elevation in right ven_tricular filling pressure, in relation to left ventricular filling pressure, is associated with renal impairment and increased mortality in advanced decompensated heart failure. Am Heart J 2015;169:806-12.

74. Lo KB, Mezue K, Ram P, et al. Echocardiographic and hemodynamic parameters associated with diminishing renal filtration among patients with heart failure with preserved ejection fraction. Cardiorenal Med 2019;9:83-91.

75. Akanksha Agrawal, Mario Naranjo, Napatt Kanjanahattakij, Janani Rangaswami, Shuchita, Cardiorenal syndrome in heart failure with preserved ejection fraction-an under-recognized clinical entity, Heart Failure Reviews (2019) 24:421-437 https://doi.org/10.1007/s10741-018-09768-9.

76. Winton FR. The influence of venous pressure on the isolated mammalian kidney. J Physiol 1931;72(1): 49-61.

77. Schrier RW, De Wardener HE. Tubular reabsorption of sodium ion: influence of factors other than aldo_sterone and glomerular filtration rate. 2. N Engl J Med 1971;285(23):1292-303.

78. Verbrugge FH, Dupont M, Steels P, et al. Abdom_inal contributions to cardiorenal dysfunction in congestive heart failure. J Am Coll Cardiol 2013; 62(6):485-95.

79. Konstam MA, Kiernan MS, Bernstein D, et al. Evaluation and management of right_sided heart failure: a scientific statement from the. Am Heart Associat. Circ 2018;137:e578-622.

80. Scantlebury DC, Hayes SN, Garovic VD. Pre-eclampsia and mater_nal placental syndromes: an indicator or cause of long-term cardio_vascular disease? Heart. 2012;98(15):1109-11. doi:10.1136/heartjnl_2012-30207.

81. Maynard SE, Min JY, Merchan J, Lim KH, Li J, Mondal S, et al. Excess placental soluble fms-like tyrosine kinase 1 (sFlt1) may con_tribute to endothelial dysfunction, hypertension, and proteinuria in preeclampsia. J Clin Invest. 2003;111(5):649-58. doi:10.1172 /JCI17189.

82. Craici I, Wagner SJ, Weissgerber TL, Grande JP, Garovic VD. Advances in the pathophysiology if pre-eclampsia and related podocyte injury. Kidney Int. 2014;86(2):275-85.

83   Fisher KA, Luger A, Spargo BH, Lindheimer MD. Hypertension in pregnancy: clinical-pathological correlations and remote prognosis. Medicine. 1981;60(4):267-76.

84. Valentin Maisonsa,, Jean-Michel Halimia, Gregoire Fauchier, et al.Type 2 diabetes and cardiorenal syndromes. A nationwide French hospital cohort study Diabetes & Metabolism 49 (2023) 101441.

85. Denis J. Donovan, Namrata G. Jain, Valeriya M. Feygina, Hilda E, Fernandez, Warren A, Zuckerman, novel approach to pediatric cardiorenal syndrome, Elsevier, Progress in Pediatric Cardiology 69 (2023) 101635.

86. Felker GM, Lee KL, Bull DA, et al. Diuretic strategies in patients with acute decom_pensated heart failure. N Engl J Med 2011;364:797-805.

87. Kuriyama A, Urushidani S. Continuous versus intermittent administration of furose_mide in acute decompensated heart failure: a systematic review and meta-analysis. Heart Fail Rev 2019;24:31-9.

88. Grodin JL, Stevens SR, de Las Fuentes L, et al. Intensification of medication therapy for cardiorenal syndrome in acute decompensated heart failure. J Card Fail 2016;22:26-32.

89. Rao VS, Ahmad T, Brisco-Bacik MA, et al. Renal effects of intensive volume removal in heart failure patients with preexisting worsening renal function. Circ Heart Fail 2019;12:e005552.

90. Caravaca P_erez P, Nuche J, Mor_an Fern_andez L, et al. Potential role of natriuretic response to furosemide stress test during acute heart failure. Circ Heart Fail 2021;14:e008166.

91. Ahmad T, Jackson K, Rao VS, et al. Worsening renal function in patients with acute heart failure undergoing aggressive diuresis is not associated with tubular injury. Circulation 2018;137:2016-28.

92. Ter Maaten JM, Beldhuis IE, van der Meer P, et al. Natriuresis-guided therapy in acute heart failure: rationale and design of the Pragmatic Urinary Sodium-based treatment algoritHm in Acute Heart Failure (PUSH-AHF) trial. Eur J Heart Fail 2022;24:385-92.

93. Bart BA, Goldsmith SR, Lee KL, et al. Ultrafiltration in decompensated heart failure with cardiorenal syndrome. N Engl J Med 2012;367:2296-304.

94. Costanzo MR, Negoianu D, Jaski BE, et al. Aquapheresis versus intravenous diu_retics and hospitalizations for heart failure. JACC Heart Fail 2016;4:95-105.

95. Sens F, Schott-Pethelaz AM, Labeeuw M, Colin C, Villar E. Survival advantage of hemodialysis relative to peritoneal dialysis in patients with end-stage renal disease and congestive heart failure. Kidney Int 2011;80:970-7.

96. Kawaguchi Y, Hasegawa T, Nakayama M, Kubo H, Shigematu T. Issues affecting the longevity of the continuous peritoneal dialysis therapy. Kidney Int Suppl 1997;62:S105-7.

97. Kraus MA, Kansal S, Copland M, Komenda P, Weinhandl ED, Bakris GL, et al. Intensive hemodialysis and potential risks with increasing treatment. Am J Kidney Dis 2016;68(5s1):S51-s8.

98. Kanbay M, Ertuglu LA, Afsar B, et al. An update review of intradialytic hypoten_sion: concept, risk factors, clinical implications and management. Clin Kidney J 2020;13:981-93.

99. Triposkiadis FK, Butler J, Karayannis G, et al. Efficacy and safety of high dose ver_sus low dose furosemide with or without dopamine infusion: the Dopamine in Acute Decompensated Heart Failure II (DAD-HF II) trial. Int J Cardiol 2014;172:115-21.

100. Wan SH, Stevens SR, Borlaug BA, et al. Differential response to low-dose dopa_mine or low-dose nesiritide in acute heart failure with reduced or preserved ejection fraction: results from the ROSE AHF Trial (renal

optimization strategies evaluation in acute heart failure). Circ Heart Fail 2016;9.

101. Bistola V, Arfaras-Melainis A, Polyzogopoulou E, Ikonomidis I, Parissis J. Ino_tropes in acute heart failure: from guidelines to practical use: therapeutic options and clinical practice. Card Fail Rev 2019;5:133-9.V.

102. Mebazaa A, Nieminen MS, Packer M, et al. Levosimendan vs dobutamine for patients with acute decompensated heart failure: the SURVIVE Randomized Trial. JAMA 2007;297:1883-91.

103. Lannemyr L, Ricksten SE, Rundqvist B, et al. Differential effects of levosimendan and dobutamine on glomerular filtration rate in patients with heart failure and renal impairment:a randomized double-blind controlled trial. J Am Heart Assoc 2018;7: e008455.

104. Teerlink JR, Diaz R, Felker GM, et al. Cardiac myosin activation with omecamtiv mecarbil in systolic heart failure. N Engl J Med 2021;384:105-16.

105. Gheorghiade M, Konstam MA, Burnett JC, Jr, et al. Short-term clinical effects of tolvaptan, an oral vasopressin antagonist, in patients hospitalized for heart failure: the EVEREST Clinical Status Trials. JAMA 2007;297:1332-43.

106. Konstam MA, Kiernan M, Chandler A, et al. Short-term effects of tolvaptan in patients with acute heart failure and volume overload. J Am Coll Cardiol 2017;69:1409-19.

107. Mullens W, Martens P, Testani JM, et al. Renal effects of guideline-directed medical therapies in heart failure: a consensus document from the heart failure association of the european society of cardiology. Eur J Heart Fail 2022;24:603-19.

108. Edner M, Benson L, Dahlstr€om U, Lund LH. Association between renin-angiotensin system antagonist use and mortality in heart failure with severe renal insufficiency: a prospective propensity score-matched cohort study. Eur Heart J 2015;36:2318- 26.

109. Berger AK, Duval S, Manske C, et al. Angiotensin-converting enzyme inhibitors and angiotensin receptor blockers in patients with congestive heart failure and chronic kidney disease. Am Heart J 2007;153:1064-73.

110. Yusuf S, Pitt B, Davis CE, Hood WB, Cohn JN. Effect of enalapril on survival in patients with reduced left ventricular ejection fractions and congestive heart failure. N Engl J Med 1991;325:293-302.

111. Solomon SD, McMurray JJV, Anand IS, et al. Angiotensin-neprilysin inhibition in heart failure with preserved ejection fraction. N Engl J Med 2019;381:1609- 20.

112. Lee S, Oh J, Kim H, et al. Sacubitril/valsartan in patients with heart failure with reduced ejection fraction with end-stage of renal disease. ESC Heart Fail 2020;7:1125-9.

113. Bakris GL, Agarwal R, Anker SD, et al. Effect of finerenone on chronic kidney dis_ease outcomes in type II diabetes. N Engl J Med 2020;383:2219-29.

114. Cice G, Ferrara L, D'Andrea A, et al. Carvedilol increases two-year survivalin dialy_sis patients with dilated cardiomyopathy: a prospective, placebo-controlled trial. J Am Coll Cardiol 2003;41:1438-44.

115. Wali RK, Iyengar M, Beck GJ, et al. Efficacy and safety of carvedilol in treatment of heart failure with chronic kidney disease: a meta-analysis of randomized trials. Circ Heart Fail 2011;4:18-26.

116. Kotecha D, Gill SK, Flather MD, et al. Impact of renal impairment on beta-blocker efficacy in patients with heart failure. J Am Coll Cardiol 2019;74:2893-904.

117. Packer M, Anker SD, Butler J, et al. Cardiovascular and renal outcomes with empa_gliflozin in heart failure. N Engl J Med 2020;383:1413-24.

118. McMurray JJV, Solomon SD, Inzucchi SE, et al. Dapagliflozin in Patients with Heart Failure and Reduced Ejection Fraction. N Engl J Med 2019;381:1995-2008.

119. Zannad F, Ferreira JP, Pocock SJ, et al. SGLT2 inhibitors in patients with heart fail_ure with reduced ejection fraction: a meta-analysis of the EMPEROR-Reduced and DAPA-HF trials. Lancet (London, England) 2020;396:819-29.

120. Nakhoul GN, Schold JD, Arrigain S, et al. Implantable cardioverter-defibrillators in patients with CKD: a propensity-matched mortality analysis. Clin J Am Soc Nephrol 2015;10:1119-27.

121. Pun PH, Parzynski CS, Friedman DJ, Sanders G, Curtis JP, Al-Khatib SM. Trends in use and in-hospital outcomes of subcutaneous implantable cardioverter defibrillators in patients undergoing long-term dialysis. Clin J Am Soc Nephrol 2020;15:1622-30.

122. Boerrigter G, Costello-Boerrigter LC, Abraham WT, et al. Cardiac resynchroniza_tion therapy improves renal function in human heart failure with reduced glomerular filtration rate. J Card Fail 2008;14:539-46.

123. Moreira RI, Cunha PS, Rio P, et al. Response and outcomes of cardiac resynchroni_zation therapy in patients with renal dysfunction. J Interv Card Electrophysiol 2018;51:237-44.

124. Wettersten N, Estrella M, Brambatti M, et al. Kidney function following left ventric_ular assist device implantation: an observational cohort study. Kidney Med 2021;3:378-85. e1.

125. Yoshioka D, Takayama H, Colombo PC, et al. Changes in end-organ function in patients with prolonged continuous-flow left ventricular assist device support. Ann Thorac Surg 2017;103:717-24.

126. Labban B, Arora N, Restaino S, Markowitz G, Valeri A, Radhakrishnan J. The role of kidney biopsy in heart transplant candidates with kidney disease. Transplantation 2010;89:887–93.

127. Bane O, Hectors SJ, Gordic S, et al. Multiparametric magnetic resonance imaging shows promising results to assess renal transplant dysfunction with fibrosis. Kidney Int 2020;97:414-20.

128. de Mattos AM, Siedlecki A, Gaston RS, et al. Systolic dysfunction portends increased mortality among those waiting for renal transplant. J Am Soc Nephrol 2008;19:1191-6.

129. Wali RK, Wang GS, Gottlieb SS, et al. Effect of kidney transplantation on left ven_tricular systolic dysfunction and congestive heart failure in patients with end-stage renal disease. J Am Coll Cardiol 2005;45:1051-60.

130. Hawwa N, Shrestha K, Hammadah M, Yeo PSD, Fatica R, Tang WHW. Reverse remodeling and prognosis following kidney transplantation in contemporary patients with cardiac dysfunction. J Am Coll Cardiol 2015;66:1779-87.

131 Kumar A, Bonnell LN, Thomas CP. Impact of changing renal function, while wait_ing for a heart transplant, on post-transplant mortality and development of end stage kidney disease. Transpl Int 2021;34:1044-51.

132. Gill J, Shah T, Hristea I, et al. Outcomes of simultaneous heart-kidney transplant in the US: a retrospective analysis using OPTN/UNOS data. Am J Transplant 2009;9:844-52.

133. Awad MA, Czer LSC, Emerson D, et al. Combined heart and kidney transplantation: clinical experience in 100 consecutive patients. J Am Heart Assoc 2019;8:e010570.

134. Melvinsdottir I, Foley DP, Hess T, et al. Heart and kidney transplant: should they be combined or subsequent? ESC Heart Fail 2020;7:2734-43.

135. Hedayati SS, Jiang W, O'Connor CM, et al. The association between depression and chronic kidney disease and mortality among patients hospitalized with congestive heart failure. Am J Kidney Dis 2004;44:207-15.

136. Diop MS, Rudolph JL, Zimmerman KM, Richter MA, Skarf LM. Palliative care interventions for patients with heart failure: a systematic review and meta-analysis. J Palliat Med 2017;20:84-92.

Summary

Renal failure is detected in over a third of heart failure patients. The association of these two pathologies has a poor prognosis, as it often alters the therapeutic strategy recommended for heart failure patients, and increases the progressive damage to both organs. The kidney plays an important role in the pathophysiology of heart failure, and suffers the progressive consequences of the most common causes of heart failure: ventricular dysfunction, atherosclerosis, hypertension and diabetes. Because these patients with renal failure and heart failure are often excluded from controlled trials, little is known about their optimal treatment and recommended medications. The "cardio-renal" syndrome is a hot topic, with various studies highlighting its increasing frequency and therapeutic implications. It can have harmful consequences, as it exacerbates the effects of neurohormonal stimulation, inflammation, oxidative stress and endothelial dysfunction on the structure of the myocardium, vessels and kidneys. It calls for close collaboration between cardiologists and nephrologists, and encourages prospective studies.

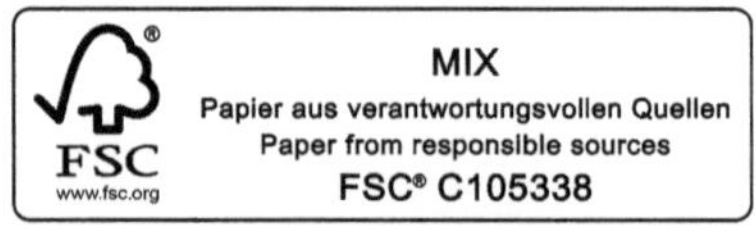

Printed by Books on Demand GmbH, Norderstedt / Germany